THE LOW CARB HIGH FAT COOKBOOK

THE LOW CARB HIGH FAT COOKBOOK

100 RECIPES TO LOSE WEIGHT AND FEEL GREAT

STEN STURE SKALDEMAN

TRANSLATED BY MONIKA ROMARE

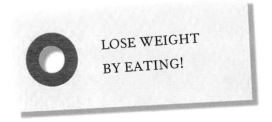

LOSE WEIGHT
BY EATING!

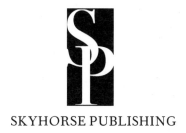

SKYHORSE PUBLISHING

I want to thank my chef friends,
Karen Pilgaard and Lars-Evert Wilhelmsson, for the wonderful recipe ideas.

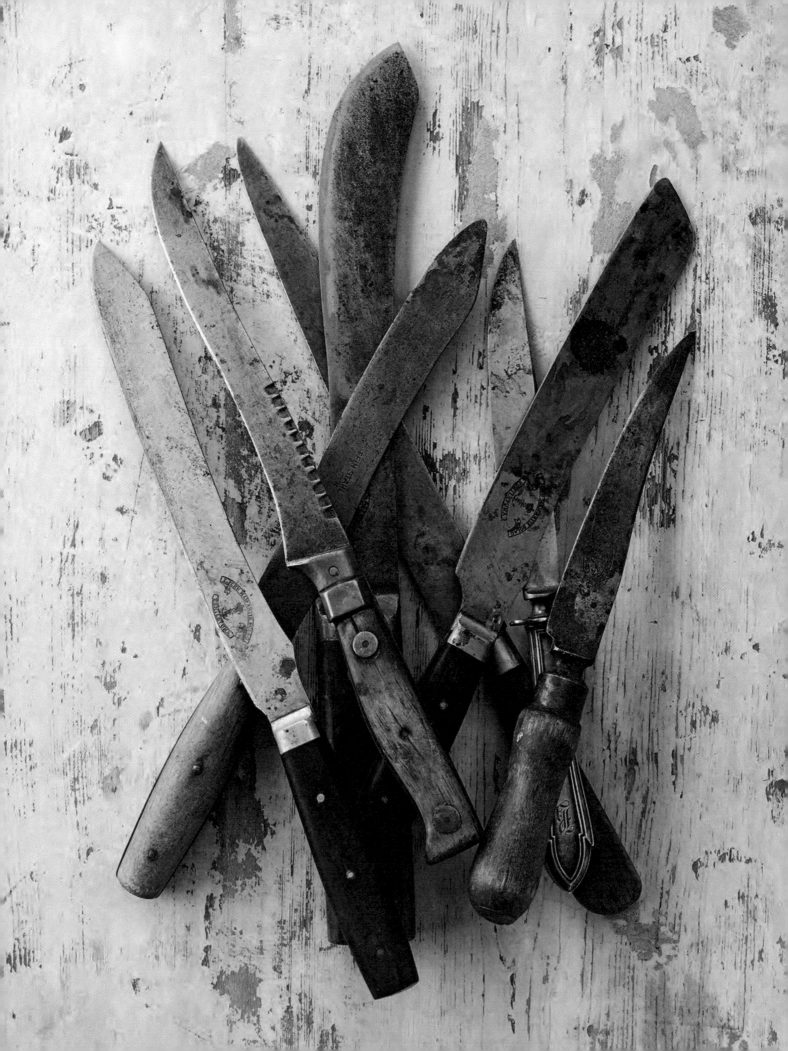

During the 1950s, when I was a little boy, nobody ever cut the fat away from ham, and most people drank whole milk. Food was home cooked, often with butter, and soda was a rarity. Fruit was scarce and seasonal. However, if you look at photographs from back then, you will discover that people were seldom overweight. Could obesity disappear if people went back to those old eating habits? Of course!

This book is about eating your way to health, happiness, and strength—without any oddities. Food shouldn't be odd. We're supposed to eat what our bodies were intended to consume, until we are full. If we follow these simple guidelines, we will feel good. If we eat food that our bodies are not accustomed to, we may become fat and sick.

Have you ever wondered why gazelles grazing grass all day long never get fat? Or why lions lazing around under the sun don't accumulate fat around the abdomen?

Is it because they exercise a lot? Or because they are calorie-obsessed? Or could it be that they walk around hungry all the time? That's what our dieticians prescribe for obesity. Eat less and run more, they say.

But lions eat until they are full and they stay in shape, even though they don't run any more than we do when we're catching the bus. Yep, they even stay in shape when they are locked in a cage. How come?

The answer is simple. Lions, tigers, gazelles, elks, and people are mammals, and they are not intended to get fat and sick. They were meant to stay in shape. The only requirement is that they eat what they were intended to consume. This book will teach you all about the foods you were intended to eat.

Sten Sture Skaldeman

P.S. I discovered the simple truth about a dozen years ago. During my first few years on a natural diet, I lost about 130–150 pounds (60–70 kg) of fat and half a dozen serious illnesses. My new eating habits made me go from unhealthy to healthy, without self-starvation or exercise. Back in the day, my ideas seemed silly to many people. Today, there are thousands of people who have the same idea of what to eat, and there is an entire movement that promotes a natural diet. I feel honored to have contributed to this movement in some way.

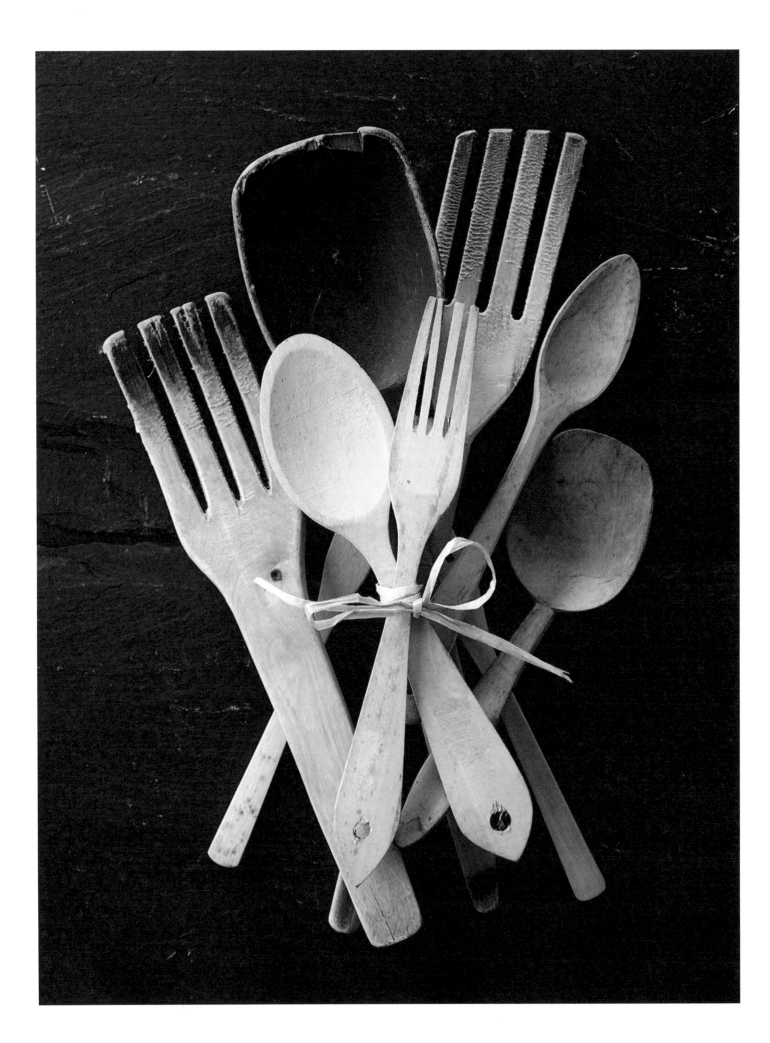

Eat vegetables with few carbohydrates!

Vegetables are a nice addition to a balanced meal. A diet that is based on animal products is the healthiest option, but we also eat with our eyes. Vegetables balance the animal portion of the meal in taste and texture, but they also make the meal look a lot more appetizing with their beautiful colors. I eat more vegetables now than I did during my low-calorie days.

Many people who have eaten their way to illness have done so with the help of carbohydrates. Most of the time, health issues that are the result of a poor diet can be eliminated by cutting back on carbohydrates and replacing them with fat. That is the idea behind the LCHF (low-carb, high-fat) diet, or what I refer to as the GI-Zero!

The easiest way to cut down on carbohydrates is to remove potatoes and grains from your diet. A small potato contains about 10 to 15 grams of carbohydrates. You should never exceed that amount of carbohydrates at any meal, and it's best if you consume even less than that. I tend to eat only a fraction of that when I want to lose weight. I do this by adding low-carb vegetables (that grow above ground) to the meat portion of the meal. Such vegetables contain less sugar and starch. Sugars and starches are carbs, and carbs slow down the fat-burning process. Root vegetables are high-starch vegetables. That means that anyone who's actively trying to lose weight should reduce their consumption of root vegetables. The only truly low-carb root vegetable is daikon. It beats every single vegetable that grows above ground. You can replace potatoes with parboiled daikon in a variety of dishes. It tastes absolutely delicious in Jansson's Temptation!

On the following page, you'll find a list of how many vegetables you can fit into a serving with 12 grams of carbohydrates. If you eat three meals like that per day, you'll stay within the daily carb limit (50 grams of carbs per day, or 10 percent of the normal energy intake).

As the list demonstrates, most people can eat pretty freely within the selection of the approved vegetables (the bottom half of the list) without exceeding a healthy carbohydrate intake. Those who have diabetes or are obese should stick to the bottom part of the list. For those people, juicy ribs, sauerkraut, and French mustard are more healing than any available prescription medicine.

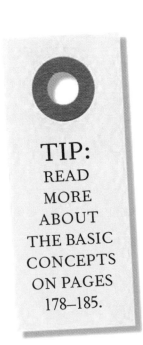

TIP:
READ
MORE
ABOUT
THE BASIC
CONCEPTS
ON PAGES
178–185.

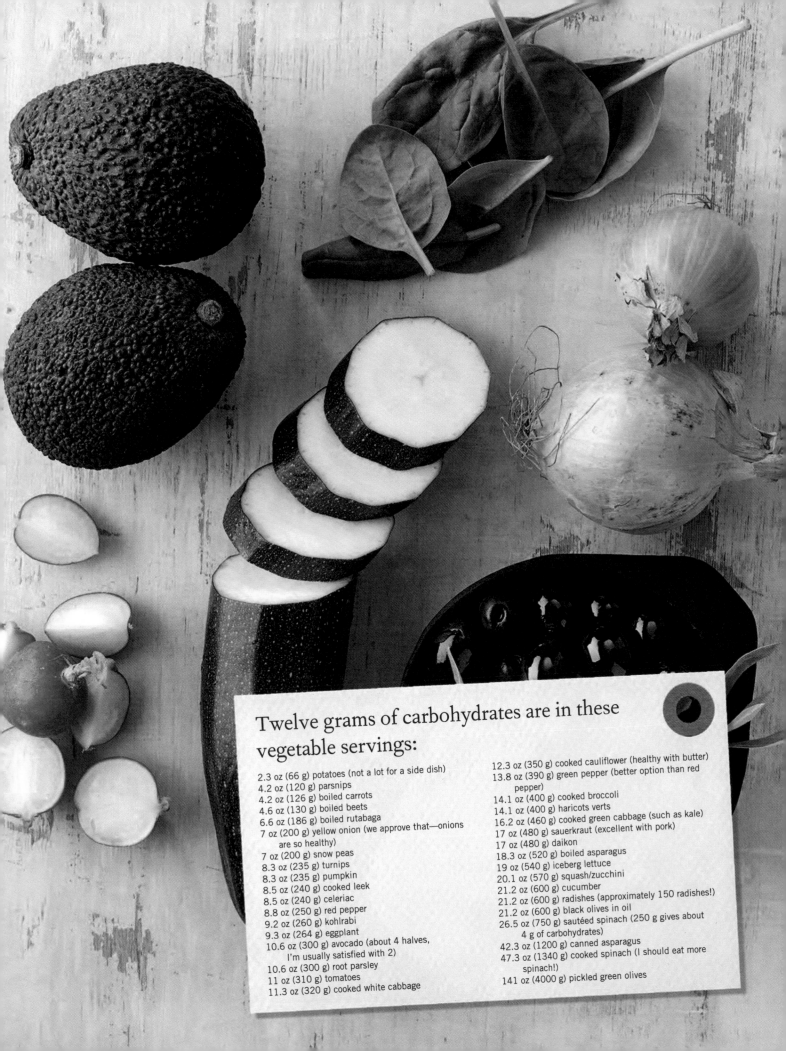

Twelve grams of carbohydrates are in these vegetable servings:

2.3 oz (66 g) potatoes (not a lot for a side dish)
4.2 oz (120 g) parsnips
4.2 oz (126 g) boiled carrots
4.6 oz (130 g) boiled beets
6.6 oz (186 g) boiled rutabaga
7 oz (200 g) yellow onion (we approve that—onions are so healthy)
7 oz (200 g) snow peas
8.3 oz (235 g) turnips
8.3 oz (235 g) pumpkin
8.5 oz (240 g) cooked leek
8.5 oz (240 g) celeriac
8.8 oz (250 g) red pepper
9.2 oz (260 g) kohlrabi
9.3 oz (264 g) eggplant
10.6 oz (300 g) avocado (about 4 halves, I'm usually satisfied with 2)
10.6 oz (300 g) root parsley
11 oz (310 g) tomatoes
11.3 oz (320 g) cooked white cabbage

12.3 oz (350 g) cooked cauliflower (healthy with butter)
13.8 oz (390 g) green pepper (better option than red pepper)
14.1 oz (400 g) cooked broccoli
14.1 oz (400 g) haricots verts
16.2 oz (460 g) cooked green cabbage (such as kale)
17 oz (480 g) sauerkraut (excellent with pork)
17 oz (480 g) daikon
18.3 oz (520 g) boiled asparagus
19 oz (540 g) iceberg lettuce
20.1 oz (570 g) squash/zucchini
21.2 oz (600 g) cucumber
21.2 oz (600 g) radishes (approximately 150 radishes!)
21.2 oz (600 g) black olives in oil
26.5 oz (750 g) sautéed spinach (250 g gives about 4 g of carbohydrates)
42.3 oz (1200 g) canned asparagus
47.3 oz (1340 g) cooked spinach (I should eat more spinach!)
141 oz (4000 g) pickled green olives

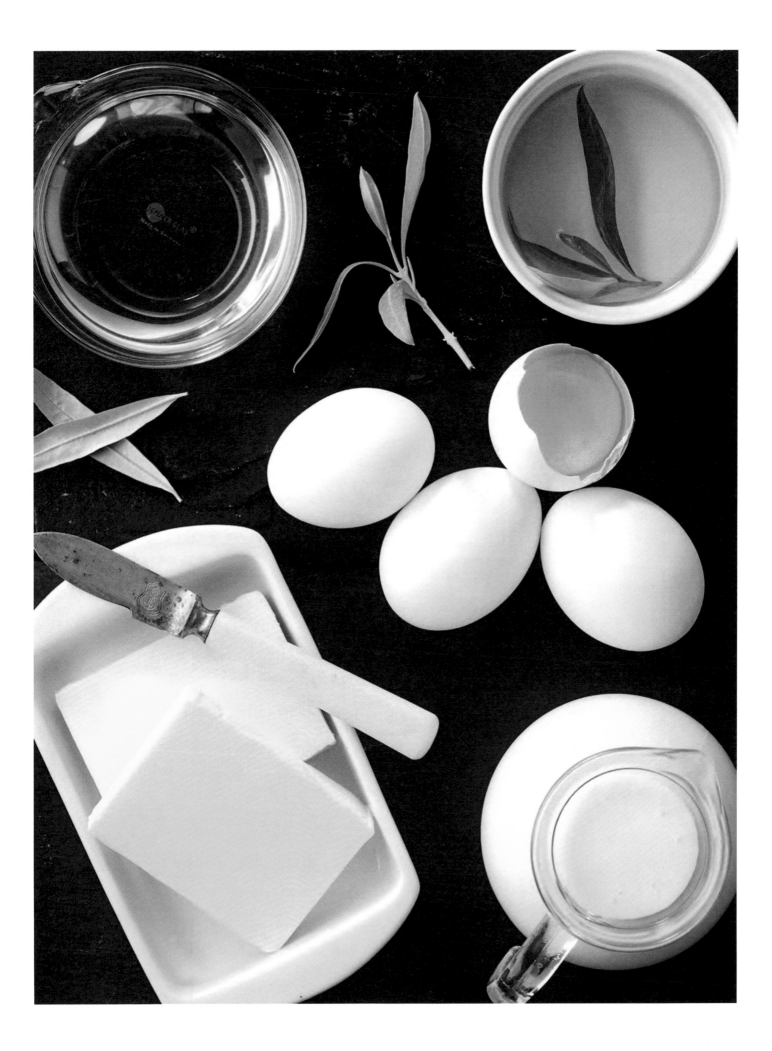

Choose healthy fats

Study the photograph. It shows you which fats to use. That's really all you need to know, no explanation necessary.

You should always use natural fats when you cook. Natural fats strengthen the immune system and protect against cardiovascular diseases. I mostly use butter. I always keep it in a bowl (with a lid) on the counter. The only reason to store butter in the fridge is if you are going to slice it with a cheese slicer over a meal.

Butter is delicious. It has been used for many centuries, and it is completely safe. Another good animal fat to complement your dishes is bacon fat. I usually have some handy in the frying pan because I cook bacon quite often, but rarely clean the frying pan. Try sautéing fish in bacon fat; the result is absolutely delectable! A century ago, people used butter, frying fat, or tallow in their cooking. There were no heart attacks back then. You can order suet at your local grocery store. Three parts ground meat and one part suet is an optimal combination for making healthy patties.

The most important fats for your health are the ones that can be found naturally in produce. Naturally occurring fat is always a better choice than any kind of added fat. The simplest principle behind cooking healthy is to choose high-fat produce and sauté the food in butter!

Natural fats are healthy fats. Unfortunately today, it is difficult to obtain all the natural fats that our ancestors had access to, and therefore we should complement our diet with natural fats from other parts of the world.

What kind of fats should we consume? Butter, coconut oil, and olive oil are staple fats in my kitchen. They are guaranteed to be healthy and have been safely consumed for thousands of years. Naturally occurring fat in meat has been consumed for millions of years. Margarine and other polyunsaturated fats, on the other hand, do not have the same track record.

When it comes to salad dressing, I base it on olive oil or mayonnaise. If I cook food over low heat, I use butter. It adds a delicious flavor that doesn't compare to anything else. When I sauté a nice piece of meat, I use butter and olive oil, or butter and coconut oil. Then I'll get a perfect combination that is resistant to high heat.

Bacon fat and tallow are two other excellent alternatives. They are perfect for pan-frying food, and bacon fat adds a delicious flavor. Cream, egg yolks, and high-fat, soured milk products are also good options. No need for any other fats.

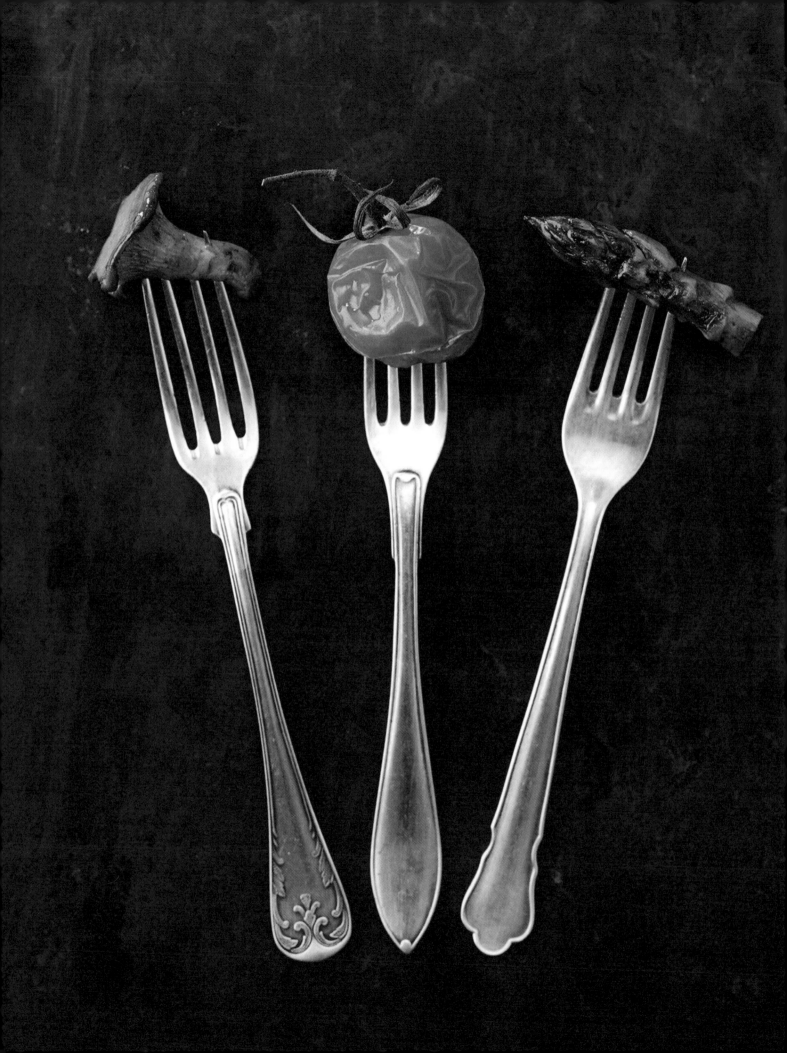

Starters

Soups,
salads, egg dishes,
and breakfast

2.

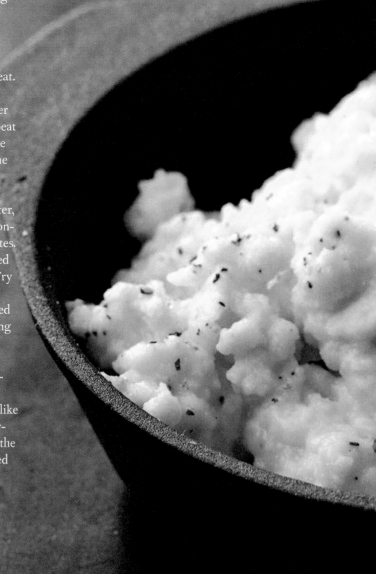

Three Quick Breakfast Dishes!

Breakfast is the least of my problems, but it's the hardest adjustment for many people starting a healthy diet. Traditionally, a Western breakfast—the kind that leads to diabetes and obesity—is based on sugar. Anything from bread and jam, to cereal, muesli, fruit, and juice.

I often get asked about breakfast. What do I eat, how much, and when? And how do I have time to cook breakfast in the morning? Well, my answer is simple. I eat a breakfast based on animal-source foods until I've satisfied my hunger, and my breakfast is usually made in a matter of minutes. Lately, scrambled eggs with various additions have graced my breakfast menu. During the summer, I tend to throw together a dish with shrimp, mayo, crème fraiche, lemon, and top it off with an egg.

1. Scrambled eggs

Heat a heavy-bottomed pan on the stove over low heat. Add 1 tablespoon of butter, then crack the eggs you will be using into the pan. Season with salt and pepper and add a splash of heavy whipping cream. Lightly beat the egg batter with a whisk. Stir occasionally until the scrambled eggs have the right consistency. I add some extra fresh pepper towards the end.

A small egg scramble made with 1 tablespoon of butter, 2 eggs, and 1 tablespoon of heavy whipping cream contains about 380 calories and 2.4 grams of carbohydrates. Fat-burning quotient: 1.6. Complement the scrambled eggs with any animal-derived food of your choice. Try leftovers from dinner—then you'll get a more balanced and nutritious meal that will keep you energized for longer. Add another tablespoon of heavy whipping cream to increase the fat-burning quotient.

I love my scrambled eggs with 3.5 oz (100 g) of cold-smoked salmon and half an avocado. Garnish with a lemon slice and some parsley, and *voilà*! A breakfast like that contains about 748 calories, and 7.2 grams of carbohydrates. This meal provides you with more than the daily recommended value of cholesterol and saturated fat, and it boosts you with vitamins and minerals. A great and healthy way to start your day!

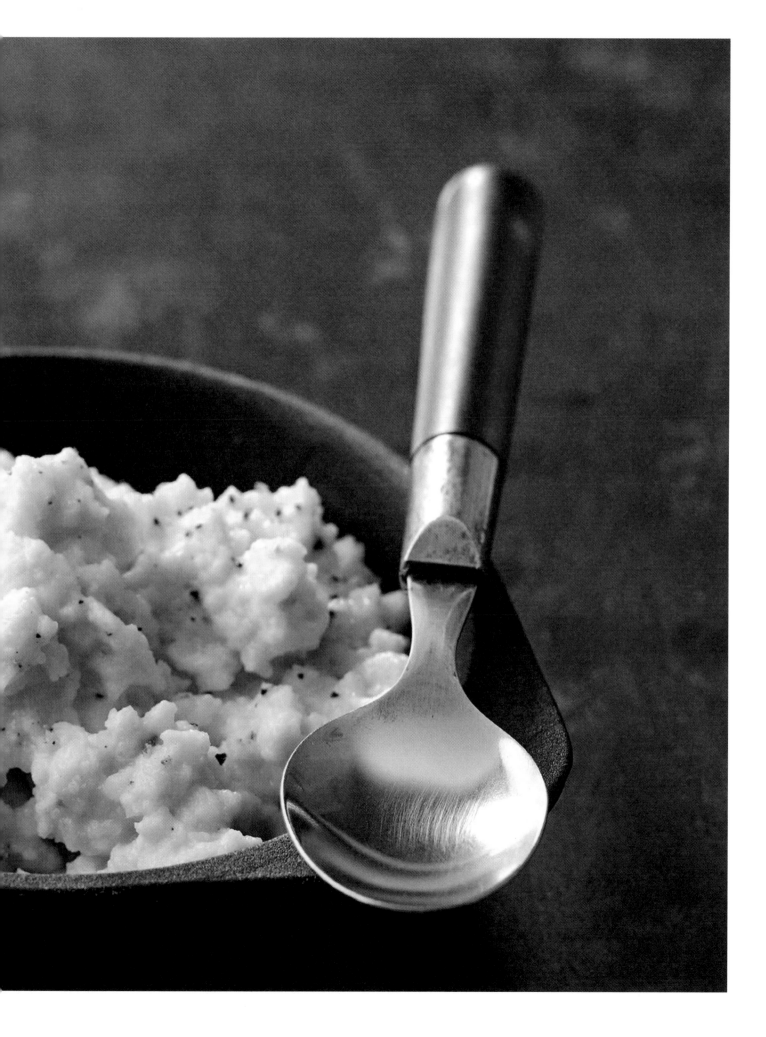

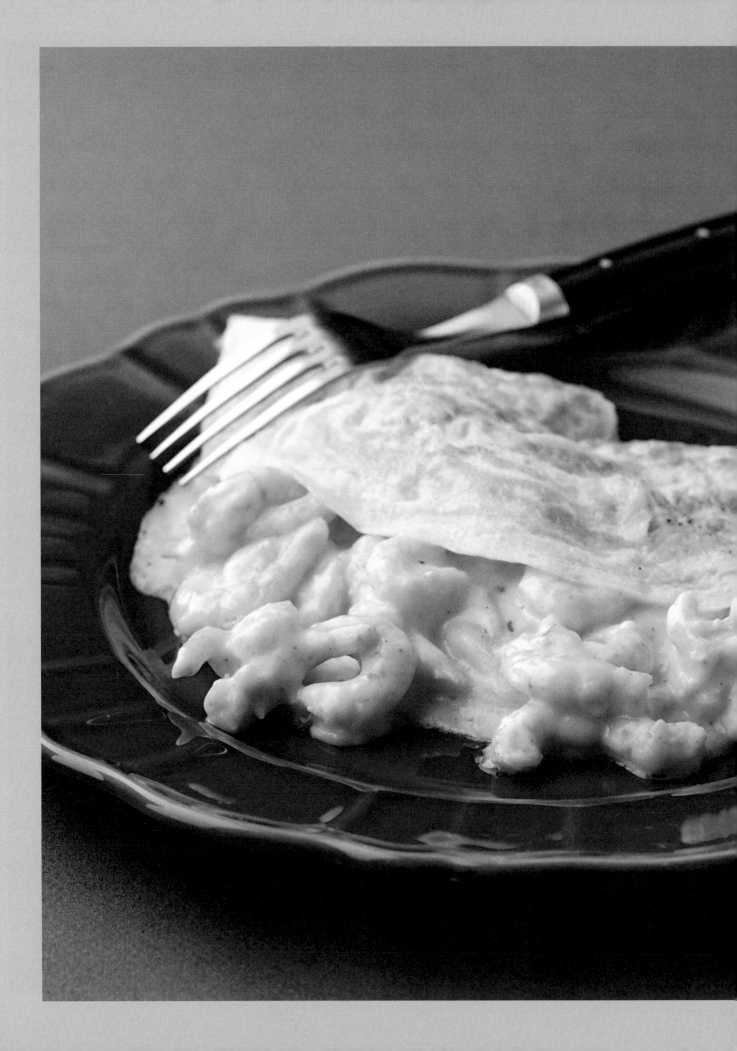

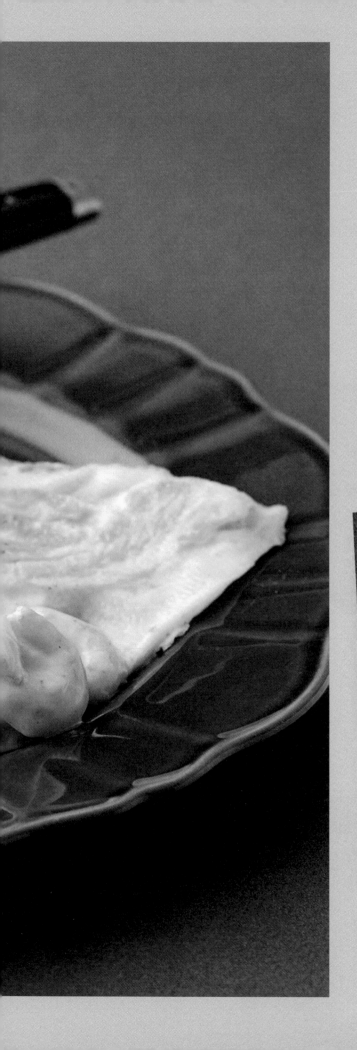

2. Quick shrimp omelet

Melt some butter in a frying pan and beat approximately 3 eggs, 2 tablespoons heavy whipping cream, 1 tablespoon water, salt, and pepper into the pan. Personally, I like to add ½ teaspoon *sambal oelek*.

While the omelet is cooking, mix some shrimp with 1 tablespoon mayonnaise, 2 tablespoons crème fraiche, and 2 tablespoons yogurt with 10 percent fat content. Try mixing in some curry for extra flavor. Place the shrimp mix on top of the omelet and fold it in half. Enjoy!

Eat half of the omelet for breakfast, and save the other half for your lunch box. One serving contains 450 calories, 22 grams of protein, 38 grams of fat, and 4 grams of carbohydrates. The fat-burning quotient is 1.5. Enough food for a petite woman. A normal-sized tomato adds about 2 grams of carbohydrates.

TIP!

The quickest breakfast is made from leftovers from the previous dinner. It is an excellent option for anyone who doesn't like to cook in the morning.

I love a couple of cold chicken thighs in the morning, or a nice minute steak stuffed with cheese. If I'm not hungry, I'll just grab a cup of coffee and 3.5 oz (1 hg) of my fat reserve, which provides about 700 calories, and that is more than enough until lunch time. However, in order for that type of breakfast to work for you, you need to be fat-fueled. By that I mean that you should have been eating a low-carb, high-fat diet long enough for your body to have gotten used to using its own fat reserves as energy. That kind of adjustment can take a few months. If you're still sugar-fueled and skip breakfast, chances are there'll be a muffin close at hand by 10 AM…

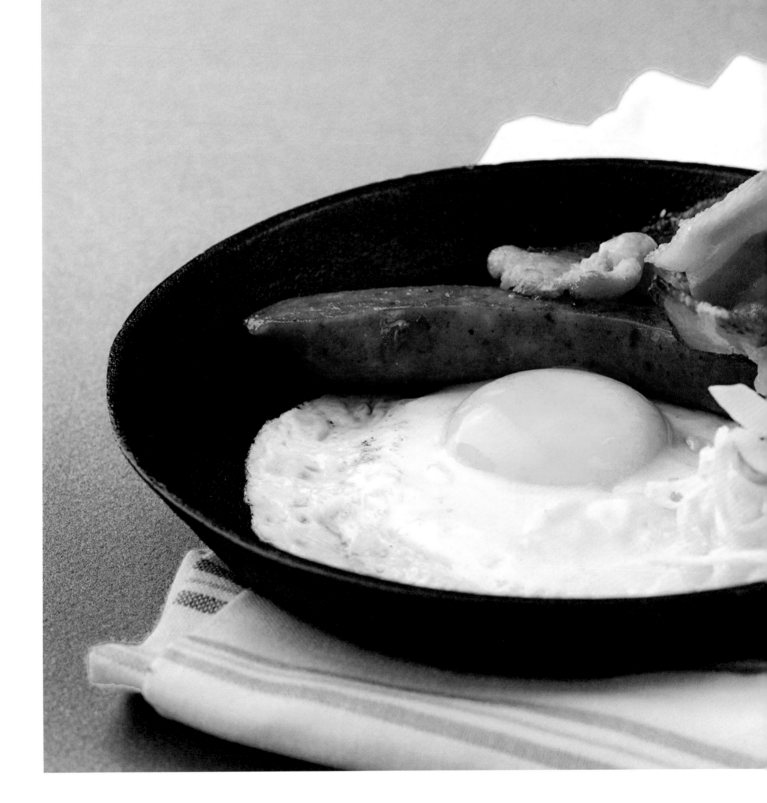

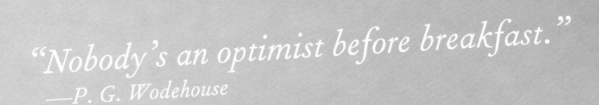

"Nobody's an optimist before breakfast."
—P. G. Wodehouse

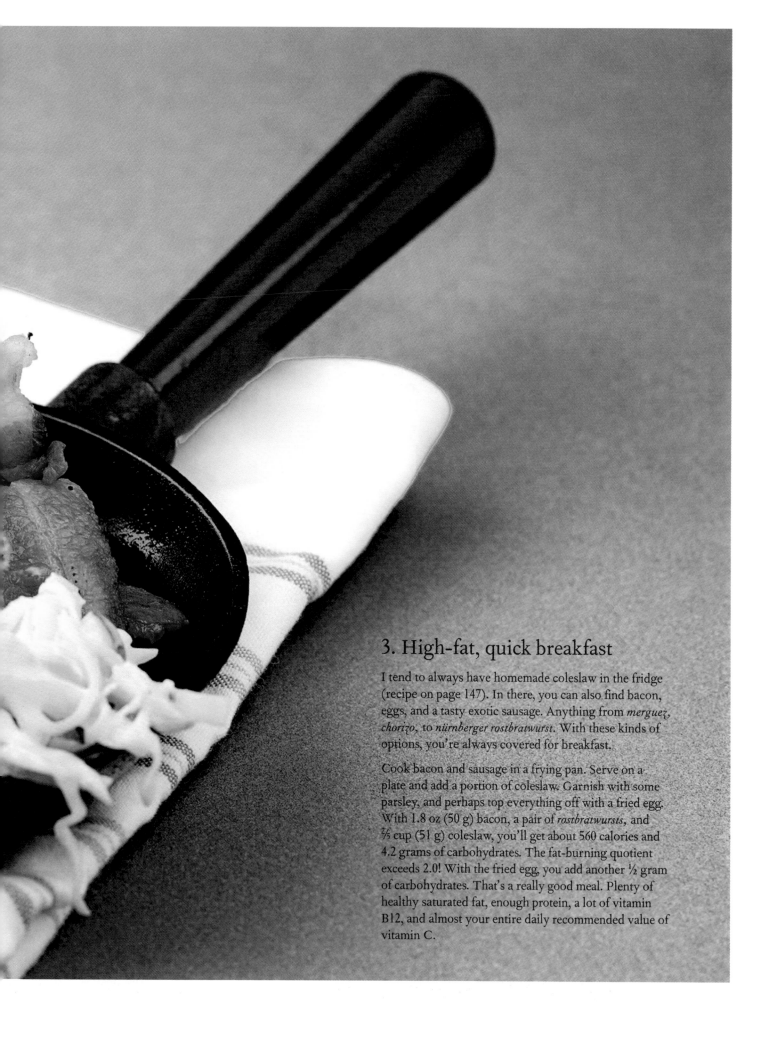

3. High-fat, quick breakfast

I tend to always have homemade coleslaw in the fridge (recipe on page 147). In there, you can also find bacon, eggs, and a tasty exotic sausage. Anything from *merguez*, *chorizo*, to *nürnberger rostbratwurst*. With these kinds of options, you're always covered for breakfast.

Cook bacon and sausage in a frying pan. Serve on a plate and add a portion of coleslaw. Garnish with some parsley, and perhaps top everything off with a fried egg. With 1.8 oz (50 g) bacon, a pair of *rostbratwursts*, and ⅖ cup (51 g) coleslaw, you'll get about 560 calories and 4.2 grams of carbohydrates. The fat-burning quotient exceeds 2.0! With the fried egg, you add another ½ gram of carbohydrates. That's a really good meal. Plenty of healthy saturated fat, enough protein, a lot of vitamin B12, and almost your entire daily recommended value of vitamin C.

Goulash Soup
Find the recipe on page 26.

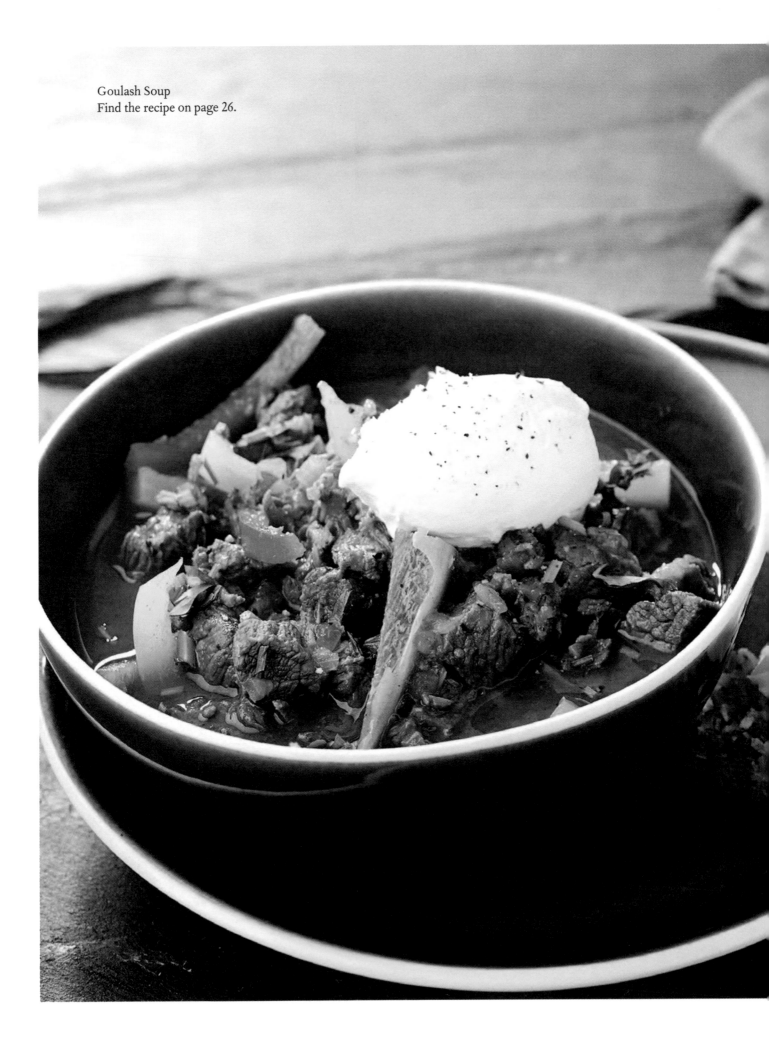

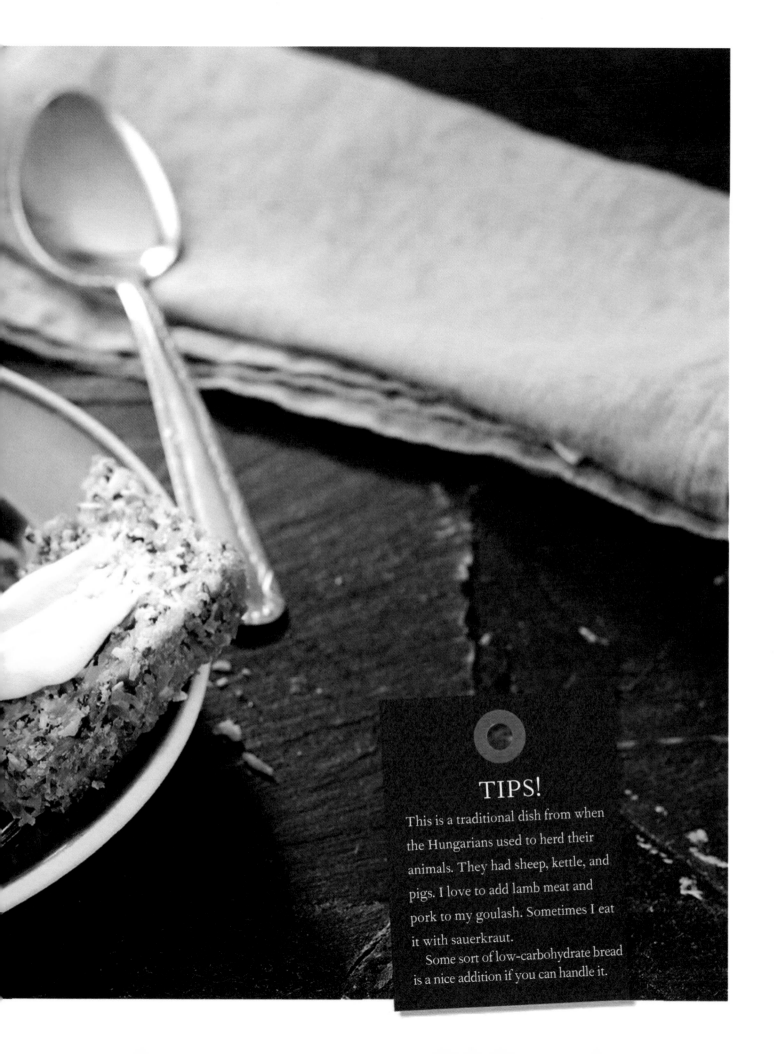

TIPS!

This is a traditional dish from when the Hungarians used to herd their animals. They had sheep, kettle, and pigs. I love to add lamb meat and pork to my goulash. Sometimes I eat it with sauerkraut.

Some sort of low-carbohydrate bread is a nice addition if you can handle it.

Goulash soup

See photo on page 24.

Goulash is usually served as a stew, but in Hungary, it is normally a soup. The only difference is how much liquid you add.

Goulash gets its specific flavor from peppers and paprika powder. Other than that, it is much like a traditional meat stew. This stew/soup is usually served with crème fraiche.

2.2 lbs (1 kg) beef, cubed

9 cups (2 liters) water/broth

Butter/olive oil to brown the meat, or lard if you are Hungarian!

2 yellow onions (about 3.5 oz/100 g)

3–4 garlic cloves, if you like garlic

3–4 peppers, preferably in various colors (about 10 oz/300 g)

1–2 teaspoons sambal oelek (I add more)

1 tablespoon paprika powder

1–2 teaspoons caraway seeds (if you want to be traditional)

Tomato purée, according to your own preference; at least 2 tablespoons

Chopped parsley (I use a lot)

Lemon zest (can be left out)

Crème fraiche

In a skillet, rapidly brown the meat in portions, transfer to a pot, and add water/broth.

Add finely chopped onions and spices. Cover and simmer until the meat is very tender and the onions are translucent. It takes about 3 hours.

At the end, add the peppers (cut into strips) and chopped parsley. Add the tomato purée. Add the lemon zest if you are using it. If you want, add more spices.

Serve smoking hot with some crème fraiche and chopped parsley.

One portion contains about 600 calories and 8 grams of carbohydrates. The fat-burning quotient is 1.

Asparagus soup is simple and delicious

If you happen to boil asparagus in lightly salted water with a little bit of butter—don't discard the water. Even if you're going to use the asparagus for another dish, the leftover liquid has such a rich flavor that it will make an excellent soup base.

Asparagus (I use about half a bunch for each person. That's enough to flavor the liquid.)

Butter

Heavy whipping cream, at least ½ cup (50 ml) per serving

Egg yolks, 2 per serving

Lemon

A few drops of concentrated chicken broth

Salt and pepper

Cut off the bottom ends of the asparagus, chop the remaining stalks into pieces, and boil them in lightly salted water with a big chunk of butter.

Put the asparagus aside and boil the leftover liquid.

Dilute with heavy whipping cream and season with salt, pepper, and a little bit of chicken broth.

When you are satisfied with the flavor, thicken the soup with a few egg yolks that you've whisked lightly with heavy whipping cream. Use about 2 yolks per serving. Sometimes I also add some cooking crème fraiche. Heat the soup until it is barely boiling, and beat vigorously. When the soup begins to thicken, it is ready.

I tend to add a few drops of fresh lemon juice at the end and garnish the soup with a few asparagus tips.

The nutritional value will vary with the amount of butter, heavy whipping cream, and egg yolks you add. Count about 2 grams of carbohydrates per soup bowl without the asparagus. The fat-burning quotient is about 5. The asparagus adds about 3 grams of carbohydrates and lowers the fat-burning quotient to 3.

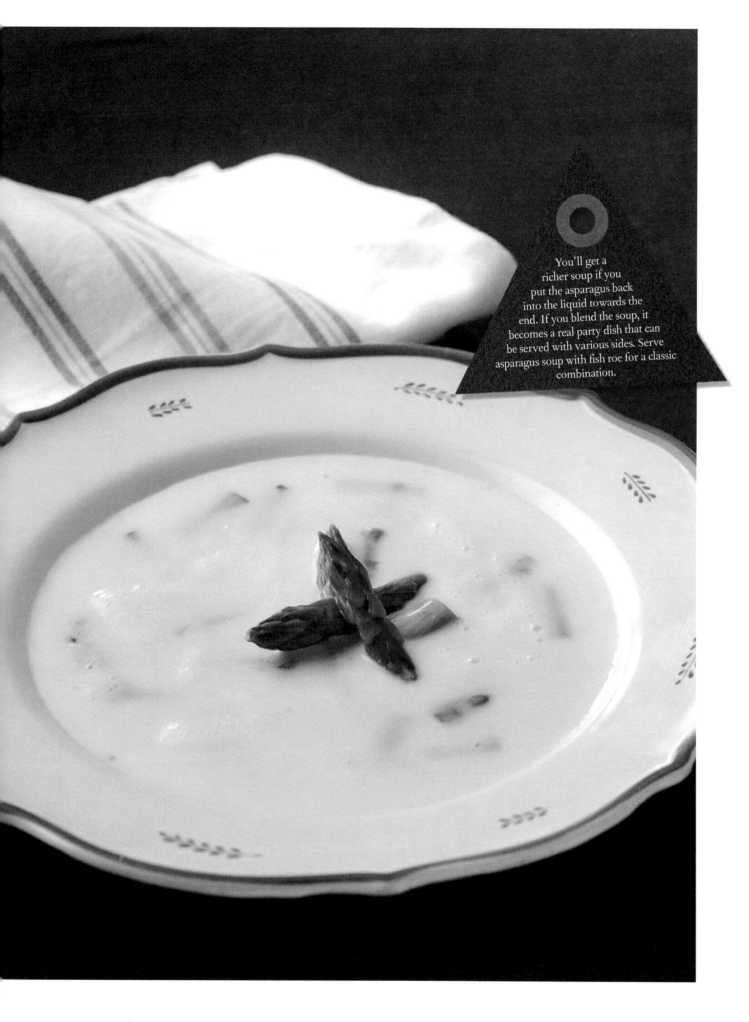

You'll get a richer soup if you put the asparagus back into the liquid towards the end. If you blend the soup, it becomes a real party dish that can be served with various sides. Serve asparagus soup with fish roe for a classic combination.

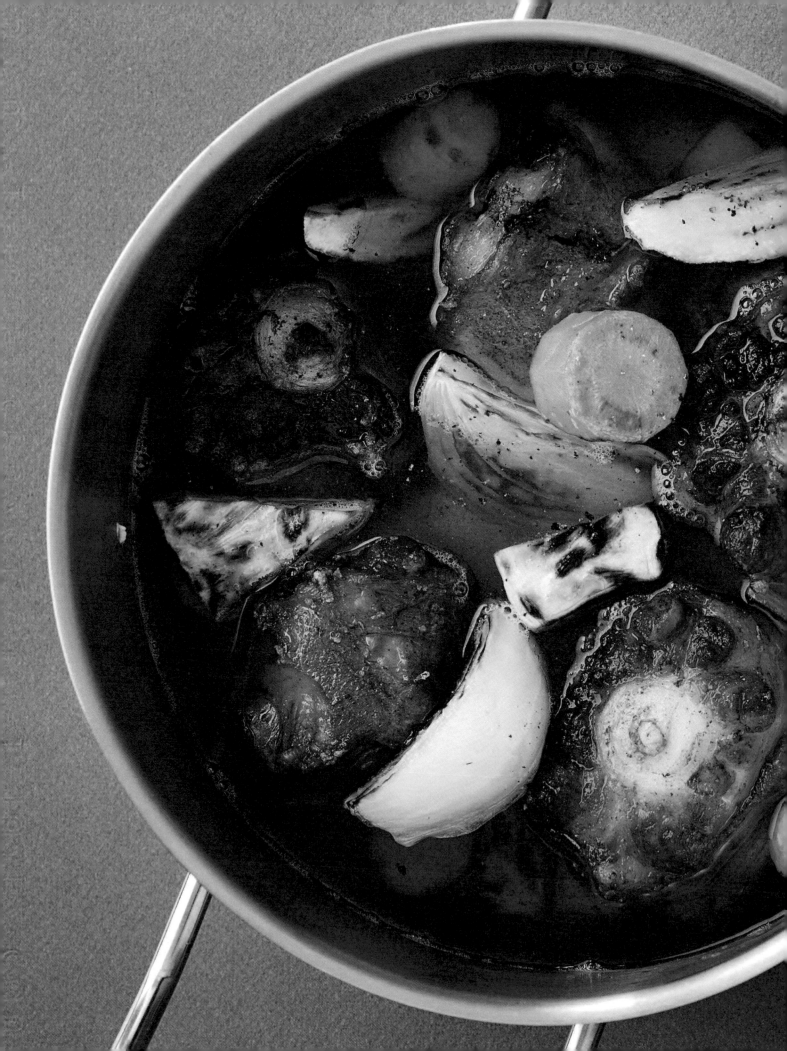

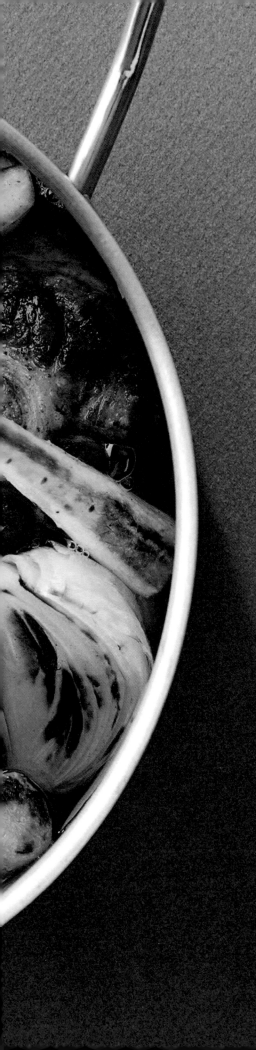

Oxtail soup

Oxtail soup is simple, delicious, and full of nutrients. As if that weren't enough, it is also very inexpensive. As with many other nutritional and affordable dishes, it requires quite some time to prepare—at least 4 hours in this case. However, you'll have plenty of time to do other things while the soup stands cooking on the stove.

An oxtail that weighs about 2.2 lbs (1 kg)

A large yellow onion

Various root vegetables, such as carrots, parsnip, and celery. If someone is very carb-sensitive, they should skip eating these root vegetables.

Cooking fat (lard is traditionally used)

4⅕ cups (1 liter) broth

4⅕ cups (1 liter) water

Spices of your choice—salt, pepper, and marjoram are common spices for this soup

Cut and clean the oxtail pieces. Brown them thoroughly in a pan.

Add the onion, and the root vegetables. Allow them to get some color.

Add the broth and water and carefully add salt. Cook until the meat falls off the bone; this takes about 4 hours.

Take out the meat pieces and remove the bones.

Strain, skim, and thicken the broth if you want. Fine chefs are very vigilant about this process. Taste and serve the thickened soup with meat. Since I always prefer to leave the fat on, I usually add the meat back into the soup, add a bit more pepper and marjoram, and serve the rustic pot on the table just like that.

This healthy dish is full of nutrients. The carbohydrate intake depends on if you eat the soup with or without the root vegetables. Count at least 3–4 grams of carbohydrates per serving without the root vegetables. The fat-burning quotient for my soup is at around 1.5. A few root vegetables add about 10 grams of carbohydrates and lower the fat-burning quotient to about 1.

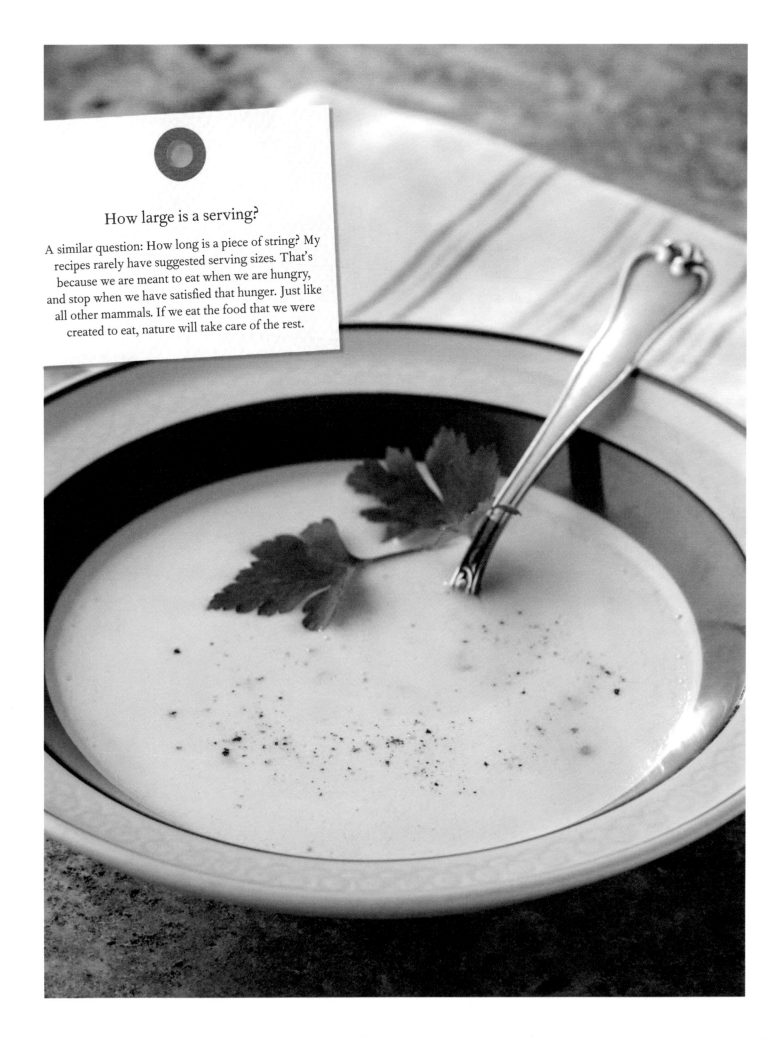

How large is a serving?

A similar question: How long is a piece of string? My recipes rarely have suggested serving sizes. That's because we are meant to eat when we are hungry, and stop when we have satisfied that hunger. Just like all other mammals. If we eat the food that we were created to eat, nature will take care of the rest.

Chicken soup

A good reason for sautéing or boiling chicken is that you can make a delicious soup at the same time! At least if you are cooking a whole chicken. If you boil the chicken, you'll use the cooking liquid as a base. When you choose to sauté the chicken, you'll make a broth from the leftovers in the pan.

For the broth:
The leftovers from a large chicken
    (preferably organic chicken)
Onion, garlic, and perhaps a root vegetable
Salt and white pepper
1 bay leaf
Fresh herbs of your choice

For the soup:

Homemade chicken broth
Heavy whipping cream, about $^2/_5$ cup (100 ml) cream per soup serving
Egg yolks, at least 1 per serving (I usually use 2 per serving)
Sambal oelek, or cayenne pepper (be careful with these spices)
Lemon

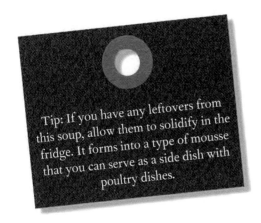

Tip: If you have any leftovers from this soup, allow them to solidify in the fridge. It forms into a type of mousse that you can serve as a side dish with poultry dishes.

Cut off the chicken breasts and thighs and place them in the fridge. You'll save them for a future dinner.

Roughly cut the remaining chicken into pieces and place in a pot with cold water on the stove over medium heat. Skim the broth once it's boiling and add the rest of the broth ingredients. Simmer for at least 2 hours. Once everything is thoroughly cooked, strain the broth through a sieve.

Now you have a nice broth that you can use in many different ways. You can cook the chicken in it, reduce the broth lightly and thicken it into a soup, or reduce the broth until half of it remains, then add cream, and you'll have a tasty sauce. Another option is to boil the broth into a fond and save it for future use. But for now, we are going to make soup.

Pour as much broth as you need into a pan, and cook it carefully. I use about 1$^1/_3$ cups (300 ml) per person. (If you have a lot of leftover broth, save it for any future poultry dishes.)

I boil away about a third of the liquid and add about $^2/_5$ cup (100 ml) of heavy whipping cream per person. The soup gets to simmer for a while before I taste it and season it if necessary. It is usually almost perfect. It is more a question about how much sambal oelek I want to add. I want the soup fairly warm in temperature, but pretty hot in taste.

Now it's time to thicken the soup. Beat some egg yolks with a little bit of heavy whipping cream. Don't let the soup boil while you stir in the egg yolks, or you'll risk getting scrambled eggs. I whisk vigorously for a minute or two and add heat until it is barely boiling. Right before the soup boils, it will start to thicken. That's when I turn off the heat and add some fresh lemon juice. Garnish with some sort of leafy herb on top; it always looks appetizing. I like to use parsley or tarragon.

Nutritional value:
One serving of soup contains about 500 calories, and about 4 grams of carbohydrates. The fat-burning quotient is 4.

A little soup lesson

What is soup? It is some sort of food, diluted with enough liquid for you to be able to eat the dish with a spoon. It isn't any more complicated than that.

Sauté nettle or spinach, and add some cream. Now you'll have a creamy sauce. Add some water/broth/wine, and you'll have a soup. Dilute a meat or fish stew, and you'll have a meat or fish soup. Many soups can be mixed in a blender, but do save some of the ingredients to garnish the soup with. Usually, you won't need to thicken blended soup.

When it comes to boiled food, you'll start with some sort of cooking stock, broth, or fond. The cooking liquid from chicken or asparagus is an excellent soup base. Thicken your soups with egg yolks that have been lightly beaten in heavy whipping cream—the traditional solution. Lightly whipped cream, crème fraiche, or crumbled feta cheese are other healthy alternatives to thicken your soup.

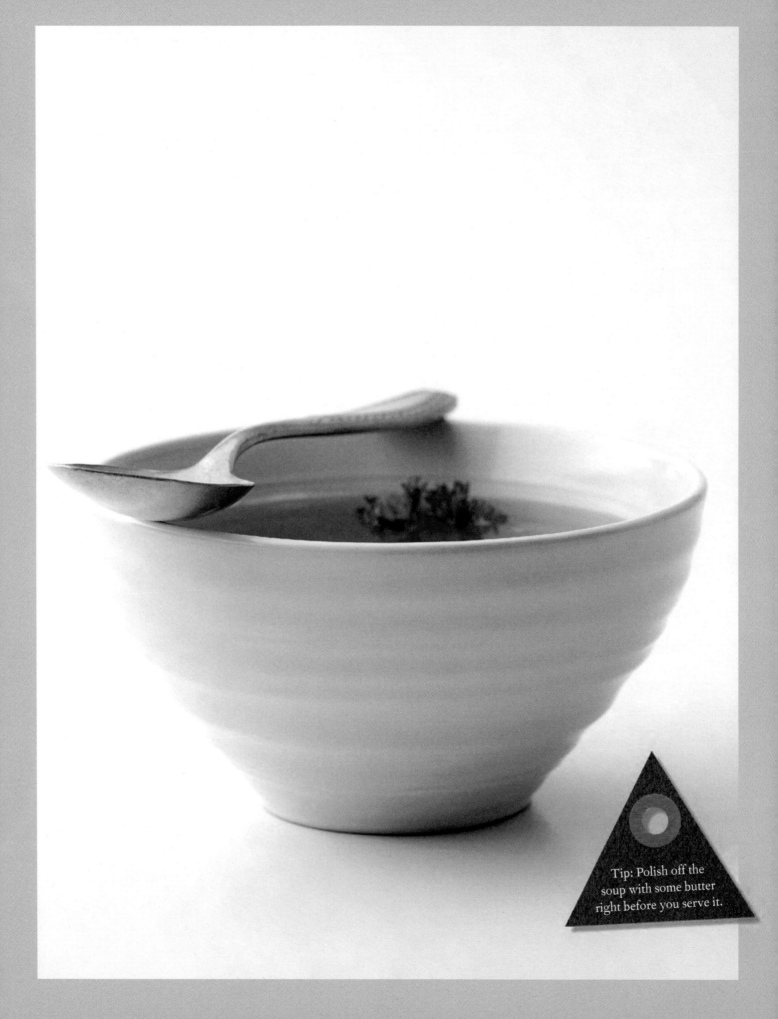

Tip: Polish off the
soup with some butter
right before you serve it.

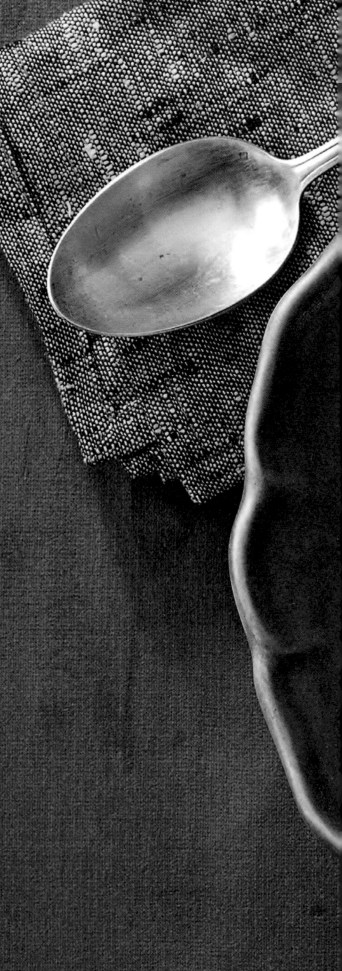

Quick fish soup

You can pretty much make fish soup out of anything, but it always tastes better if you include fish. A soup with only fish broth and vegetables is a bit plain. Keep in mind that smaller fish fillets only need a few minutes to cook! Begin by cooking the other ingredients separately and add the fish at the end.

Fish stew and fish soup are pretty much the same thing, except that the soup contains more liquid. The liquid usually consists of fish broth, preferably with a nice addition of some dry white wine. Classic fish soup recipes are usually made with an authentic fish broth made by boiling fish leftovers, but for now let's keep it simple. Let us use fish fillets (preferably a variety of different kinds of fish) and a fish broth cube.

A variety of fish fillets, about 10.5 oz (3 hg) per person
2 onions, preferably red onion or leek
1 red or yellow pepper, or anything else that will add color
A few tomatoes
A few root vegetables to flavor the soup (not for eating!)
Fish broth and/or white wine
Garlic cloves (according to your own preference)
Cooking fat to brown the vegetables—I suggest mixing a little bit
    of butter with coconut or olive oil.
Salt and pepper
Leafy herbs of your choice: Bay leaves, thyme, fennel, and parsley
    are often used to flavor fish soups. Saffron and orange zest are
    other classic choices. Use what you like.
Lemon

Coarsely chop onions and vegetables and brown them quickly in a frying pan before you transfer them to a big pot. Mix with fish broth, water, and wine. Simmer for a while before you flavor the broth with your choice of herbs and spices. Salt, pepper, and sambal oelek belong in my broth.

When it's time to serve the soup, add the diced fish, bring to a boil, and turn off the heat. The fish pieces will be ready to eat by the time you carry the pot to the table.

Tip: Fish soup is very lean cuisine, but you can fatten it up a bit by adding some cream, butter, or cheese balls that you roll out of high-fat, shredded cheese mixed with crème fraiche and cayenne pepper for extra spice. Throw a few of those balls into the soup, and you'll raise the fat content significantly. Count on about 4 grams of carbohydrates per portion once you've ridden the soup of the root vegetables. A boiled carrot will triple the carbohydrate intake!

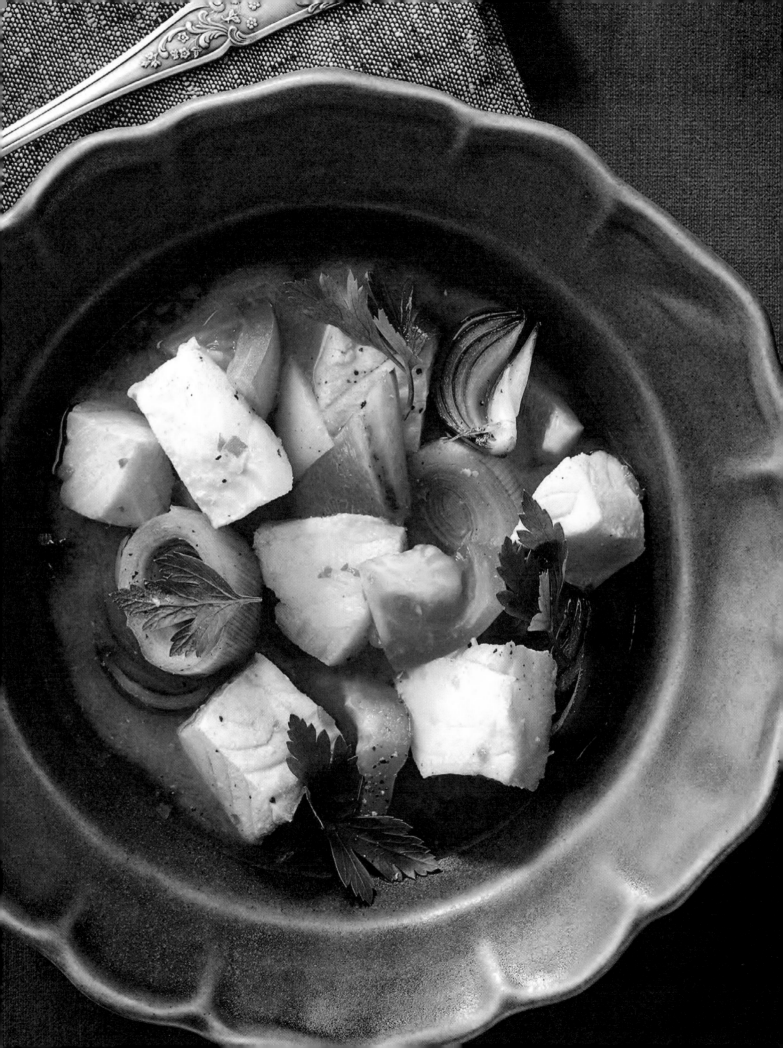

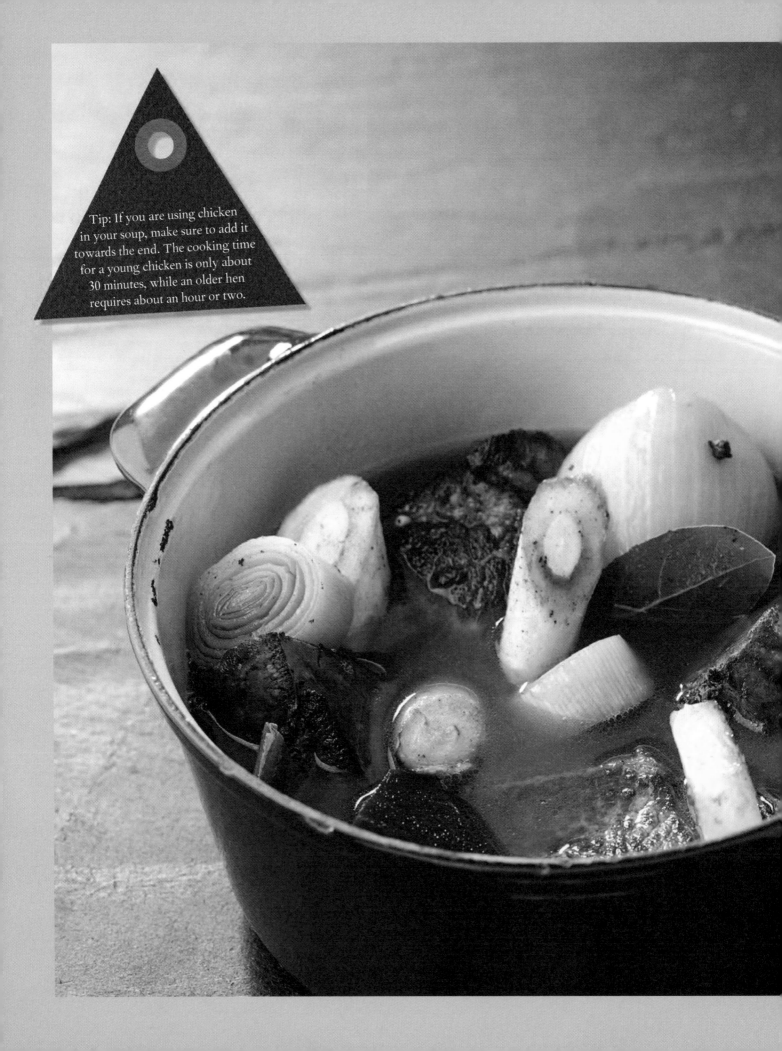

Tip: If you are using chicken in your soup, make sure to add it towards the end. The cooking time for a young chicken is only about 30 minutes, while an older hen requires about an hour or two.

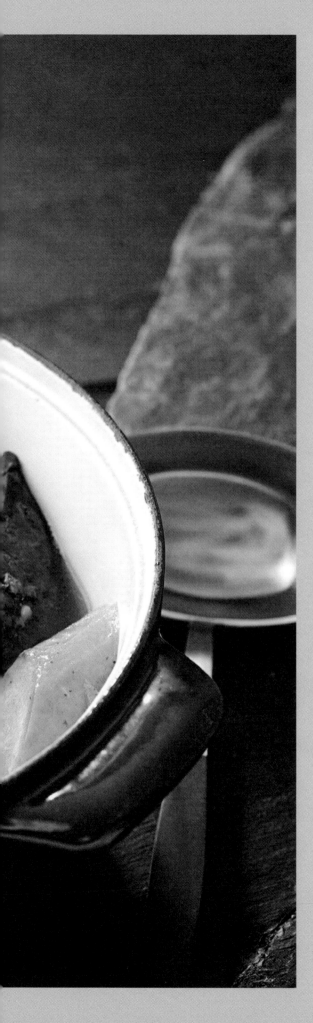

Pot-au-feu

Pot-au-feu is one of those nice French meat soups that traditionally stood on the iron stove for days. The pot would be filled with whatever was available and refilled with new ingredients as the soup was eaten. Usually, the meat and the soup were served separately.

I make pot-au-feu every once in a while during the fall. Anything except for fish tends to end up in my pot. Ox meat and marrowbone usually make up the base, but organ meats, poultry, bacon, and lamb meat also tend to end up in this dish. Together, these ingredients make a merry mix.

2.2–4.4 lbs (1–2 kg) any inexpensive chuck cut of beef

1.1 lbs (½ kg) marrowbone

3.5–7 oz (1–2 hg) beef liver (yep, it belongs in here!)

Butter

2 leeks

A few carrots and other root vegetables

Perhaps a beet for the color

2 tomatoes

Water, enough to cover the meat and vegetables entirely

2 yellow onions

1 clove (to insert into one of the onions)

Salt, pepper, and leafy herbs of your choice; Parsley should be one of them.

You can begin in two different ways:

1. Begin by browning the meat (like I always do), then add vegetables and spices and allow everything to get a nice color before you add water. Save the onion with the inserted clove for later.

2. For the French way, boil the meat in the water, skim, and add vegetables and spices. Here too, you'll save the onion with the clove for later.

Boil the soup for a few hours.

Fry the onion with the clove thoroughly before you add it to the soup.

Simmer for a few more hours. An authentic pot-au-feu should be golden brown and aromatic.

Serve the meat and soup separately if you wish to do it the French way. Otherwise, mix everything into the same bowl. After the meal, add some more meat to the pot and dilute it with more water/broth, and continue to cook the soup. If you have enough produce at home, this soup will last for a long time.

The nutritional value of this meal will depend on what you consume. Meat and broth make for a very lean dish with few carbohydrates. If you eat the pot-au-feu with the meat and vegetables, you'll consume about 4–5 grams of carbohydrates per bowl.

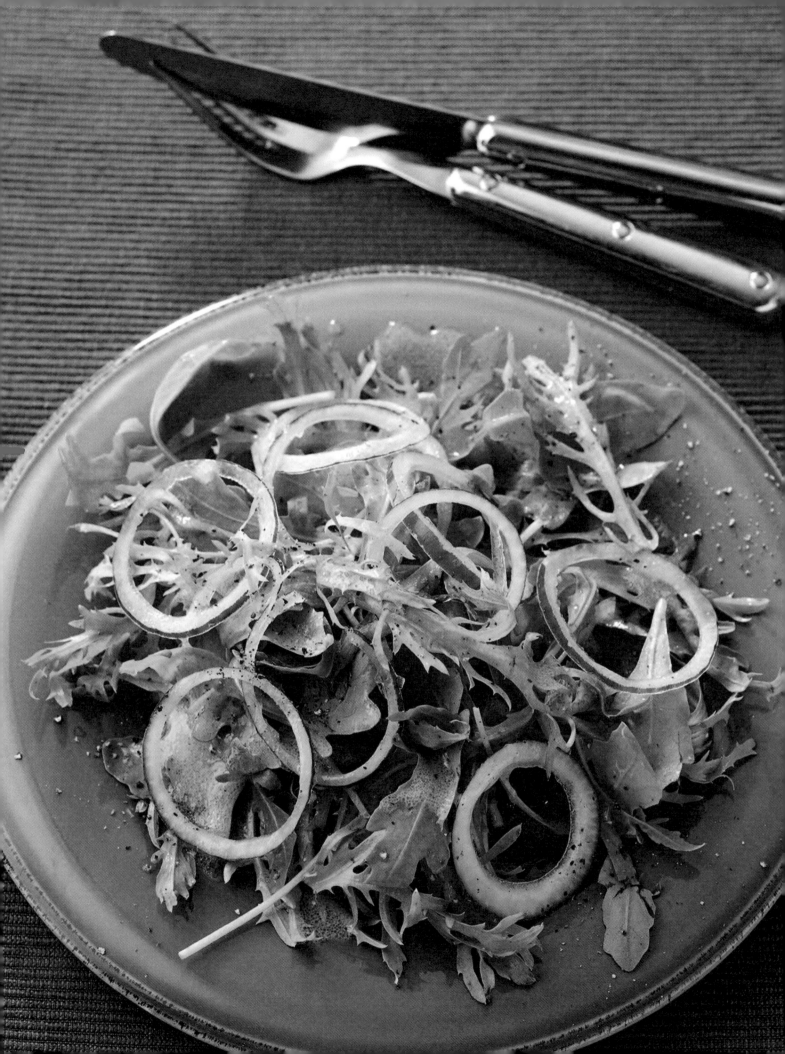

Green salad LCHF

A low-carb salad should be green. Any colorful additions usually add carbohydrates. I find the traditional Swedish salad—lettuce, cucumber, tomato, and dressing—to be pretty boring. Instead, I like to use some flavorful bitter greens, such as arugula, frisée, or fresh dandelion leaves. I spread a few thin slices of red onion over the greens and add dressing—usually vinaigrette. Top off with freshly ground black pepper, and you'll have a lovely salad!

If I want a more filling salad, I add some fried bacon and pour some of the frying fat over the salad. Then it will taste like a French salad. Fried mushrooms are another option. If I want a Greek-inspired salad, I'll skip the bacon but add avocado and olives, or feta cheese and olives. In a whip you'll have a Greek salad!

The basic green salad with greens, red onion, and dressing contains 3 carbohydrates per serving. The fat-burning quotient is about 3. With fried mushrooms and bacon, you'll get a complete meal with about 6 grams of carbohydrates, and a fat-burning quotient that exceeds 2.5.

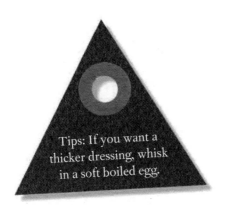

Tips: If you want a thicker dressing, whisk in a soft boiled egg.

Salad of the day (avocado salad)

Today, I began my morning by frying bacon. That's usually how I start my day. Then I took a good look inside my fridge and found boiled eggs, shrimp (in solution), avocado, and tomatoes. Naturally, there was also a jar of mayo and some crème fraiche. And French mustard. It was time for a salad. However, the avocado was hard, and the tomatoes pretty pale.

I sliced an egg and spread out the slices into an elegant arch. Then I piled shrimp in the center. One dollop of mayo and crème fraiche on the side. The presentation looked pretty decent. To top it off, I added some bacon and freshly ground black pepper. There's nothing like coarsely ground black pepper in the morning.

I skipped adding any other ingredients, and I forgot to add lemon. Despite that, the salad was delicious. Shrimp in solution tend to be very flavorful.

This simple and excellent salad only took me a few minutes to throw together. The time it takes to cook the bacon will determine how long it takes you to make it. I ate about ⅖ cup (100 g) of shrimp, a third of a pack of bacon, one egg, about one tablespoon of mayonnaise, and one tablespoon of crème fraiche. I mixed the dressing right on the plate with a fork. This salad is packed with nutrients and provides a lot of energy. You'll still feel light afterwards, but won't get hungry for another four hours.

I added this salad to my computer-based nutritional program and found that I started my day with 543 calories, 25 grams of protein, 49 grams of fat, and 2.1 grams of carbohydrates. As you may remember, the fat-burning quotient is the weight of fat divided by the sum of the weight of the carbs and proteins. 49 grams of fat divided by 25 plus 2.1 gives a fat-burning quotient of about 2. That is excellent. This simple salad provides healthy fats and it is packed with vitamin B12, vitamin E, and half of your day's worth of phosphorus and selenium.

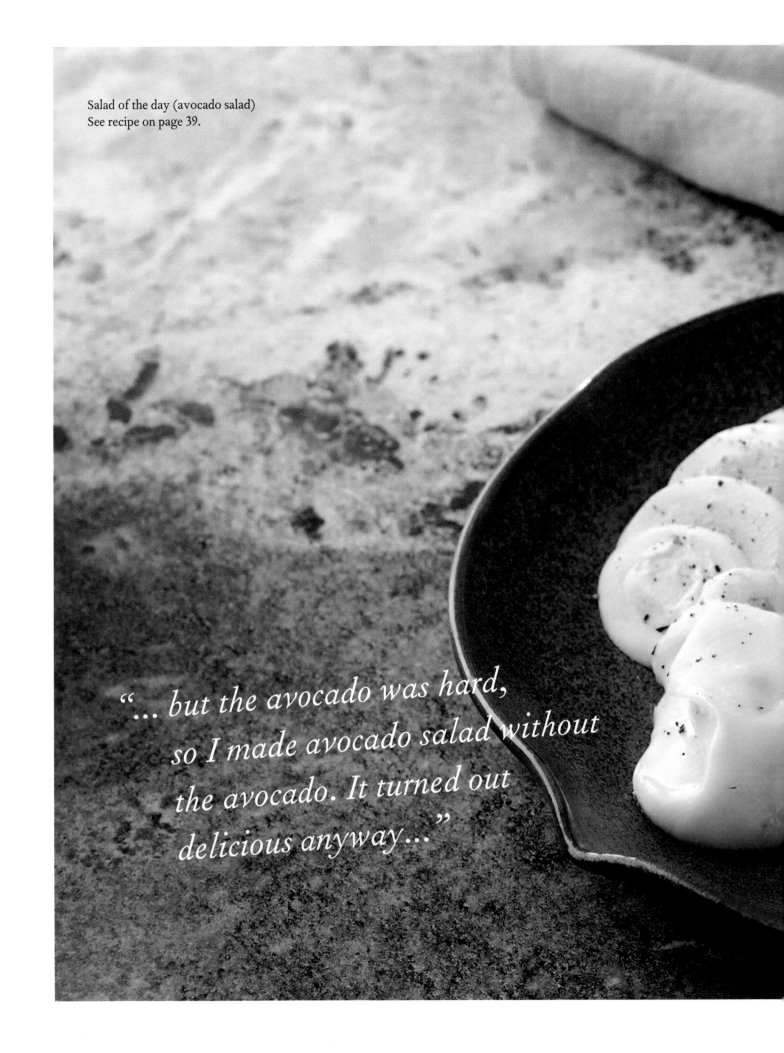

Salad of the day (avocado salad)
See recipe on page 39.

"... but the avocado was hard, so I made avocado salad without the avocado. It turned out delicious anyway..."

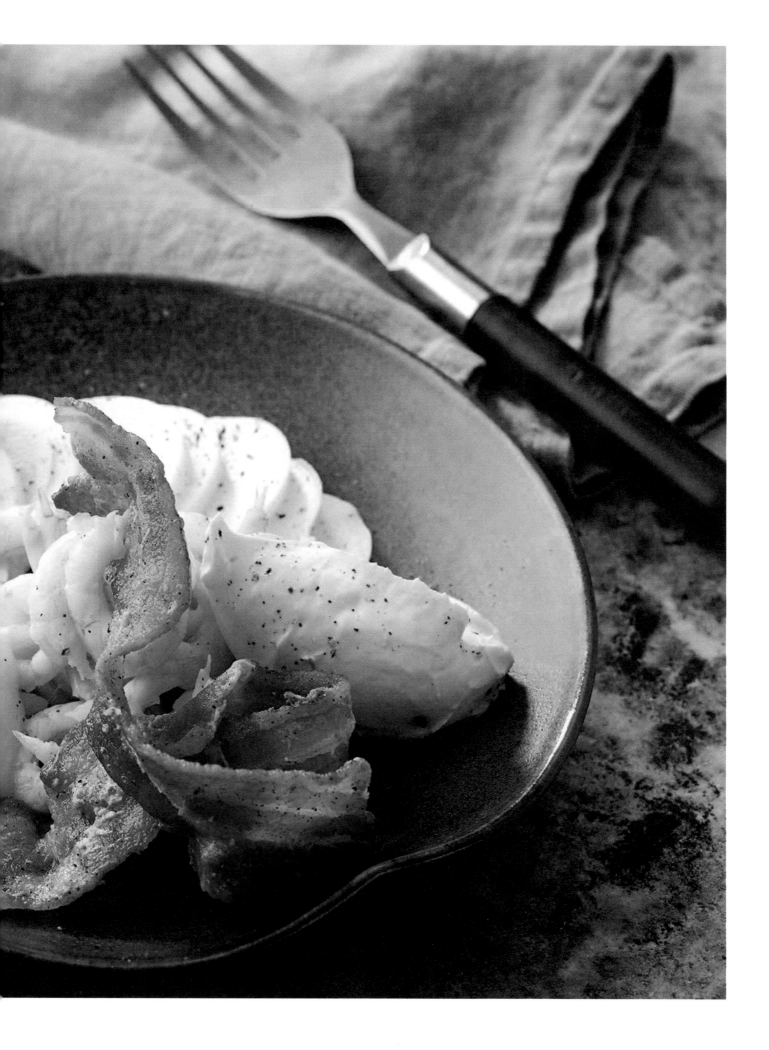

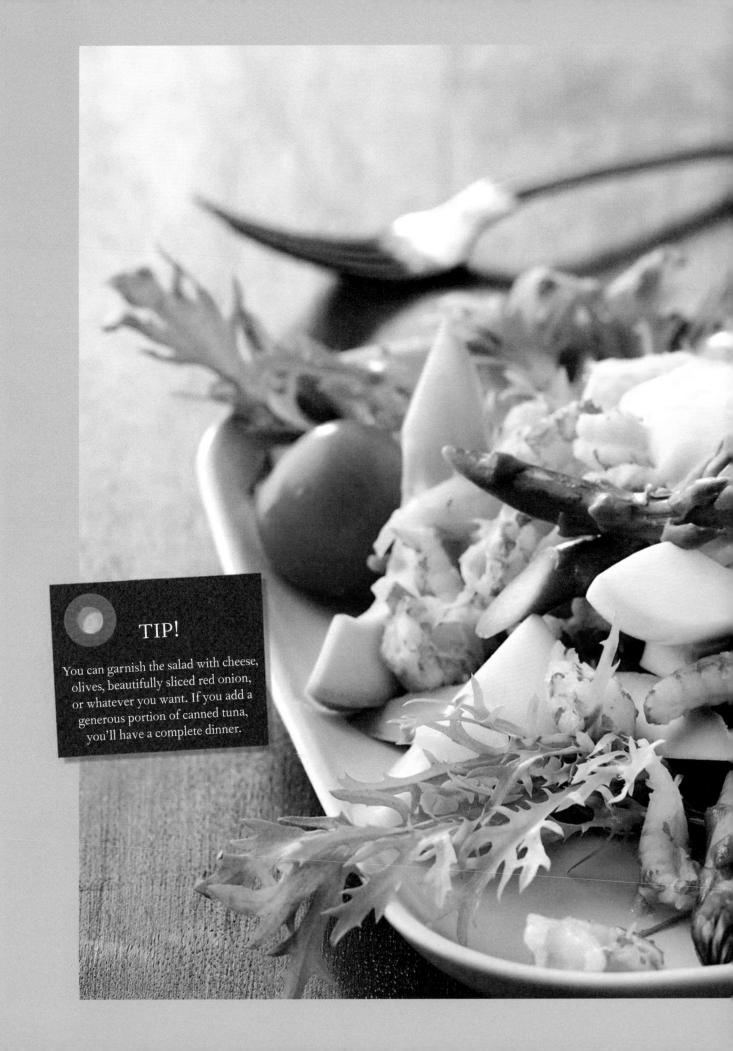

TIP!

You can garnish the salad with cheese, olives, beautifully sliced red onion, or whatever you want. If you add a generous portion of canned tuna, you'll have a complete dinner.

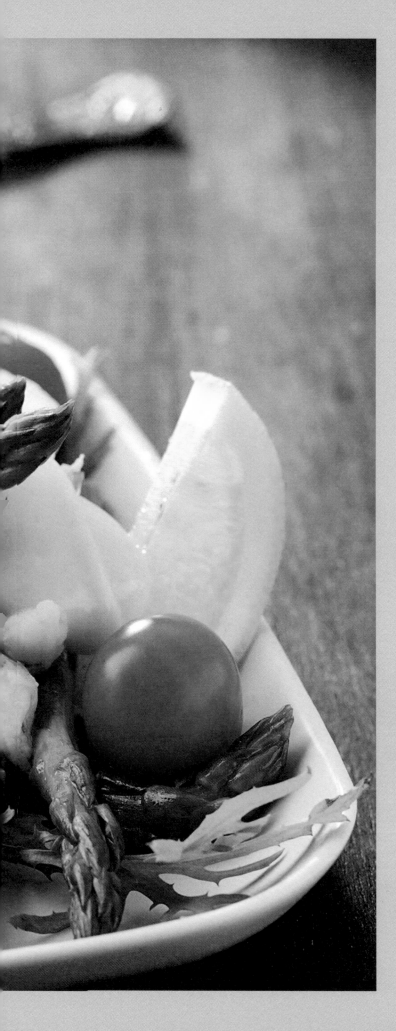

Filling salad with egg, shrimp, asparagus, and mayo

Eggs are probably one of the best things we can eat. Shrimp is delicious and packed with protein. Asparagus barely contains any carbohydrates, and we'll easily solve the fat-burning quotient by adding a high-fat dressing. This salad is easy to make and is both delicious and healthy. Garnish with a few leafy greens and a tomato wedge. You can also add half an avocado if you're in the mood for it.

½ bunch of lightly cooked asparagus (cut into pieces)

A fistful of leafy greens

½ avocado, if you want a richer salad

A few cherry tomatoes

My vinaigrette (see page 155), or lemon and olive oil

2 boiled eggs

⅖–⅘ cup (100–200 g) peeled shrimp, or crayfish tails (you can buy those in a solution)

⅕ cup (50 ml) mayonnaise mixed with ⅓ cup crème fraiche

1 lemon wedge

Parsley

Salt and pepper

Spread the leafy greens, half of the asparagus, avocado, and tomatoes over the plate. Sprinkle with vinaigrette.

Place egg halves and shrimp on top.

Add the mayonnaise/crème fraiche.

Garnish with the remaining asparagus, a lemon wedge, and parsley.

Finish off with salt and pepper.

This very filling salad will provide you with about 800 calories, and it contains about 10 grams of carbohydrates. The fat-burning quotient depends on what sauce you are using, but is usually over 1.5.

Hot asparagus salad

Asparagus is the perfect vegetable for people who want to eat healthy. Not only does it look beautiful on the plate, but it is delicious, inexpensive, easy to prepare, and it contains hardly any carbohydrates. Yes, it is almost fat-free, but don't worry—it tastes heavenly with butter, cream, and mayo.

1 bunch of green asparagus

$\frac{1}{5}$ cup (50 ml) oil

1–2 tablespoons lemon

1–2 tablespoons finely chopped onion

1 crushed garlic clove

1 tablespoon sambal oelek (it should be hot!)

Salt and pepper

Coriander and cumin, according to your own preference

Begin by cutting off the bottom part of the asparagus, about half an inch or so. Cut the remaining stalks into pieces. Boil the asparagus in lightly salted water, about one minute.

Make a dressing out of the remaining ingredients. Place the warm asparagus in the dressing, mix it in, and allow to cool. This salad goes with mostly anything, but is especially tasty with pork. Count about 4 grams of carbohydrates per serving. The fat-burning quotient is approximately 3.

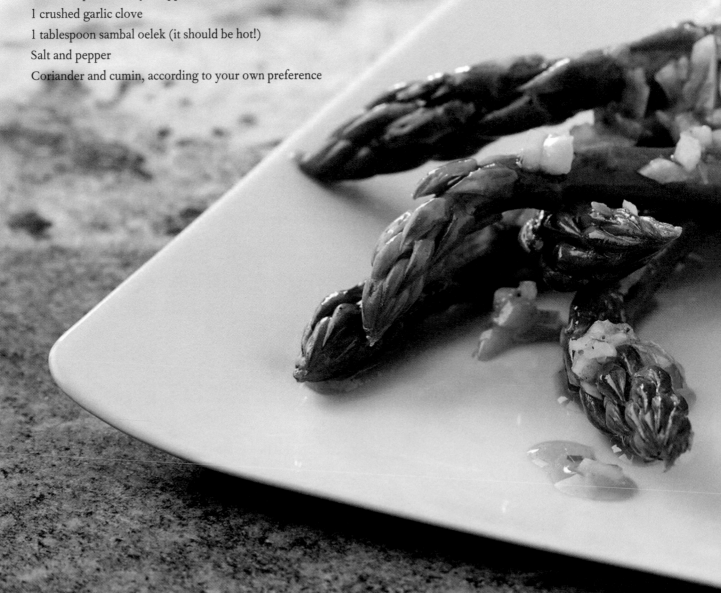

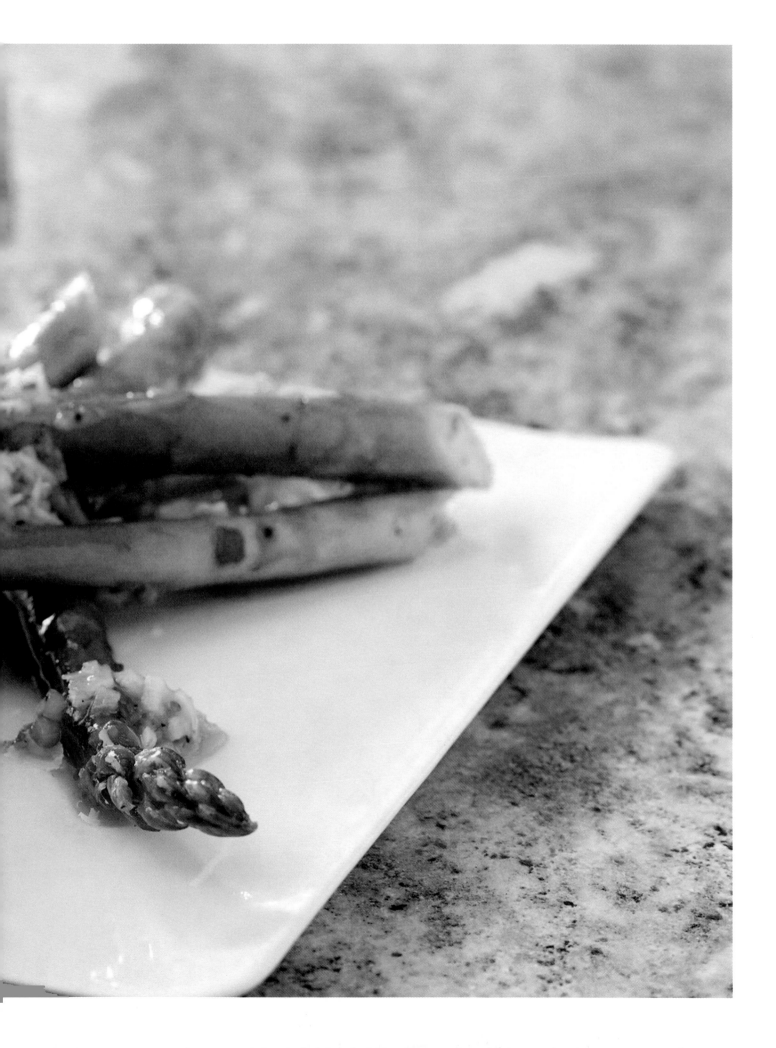

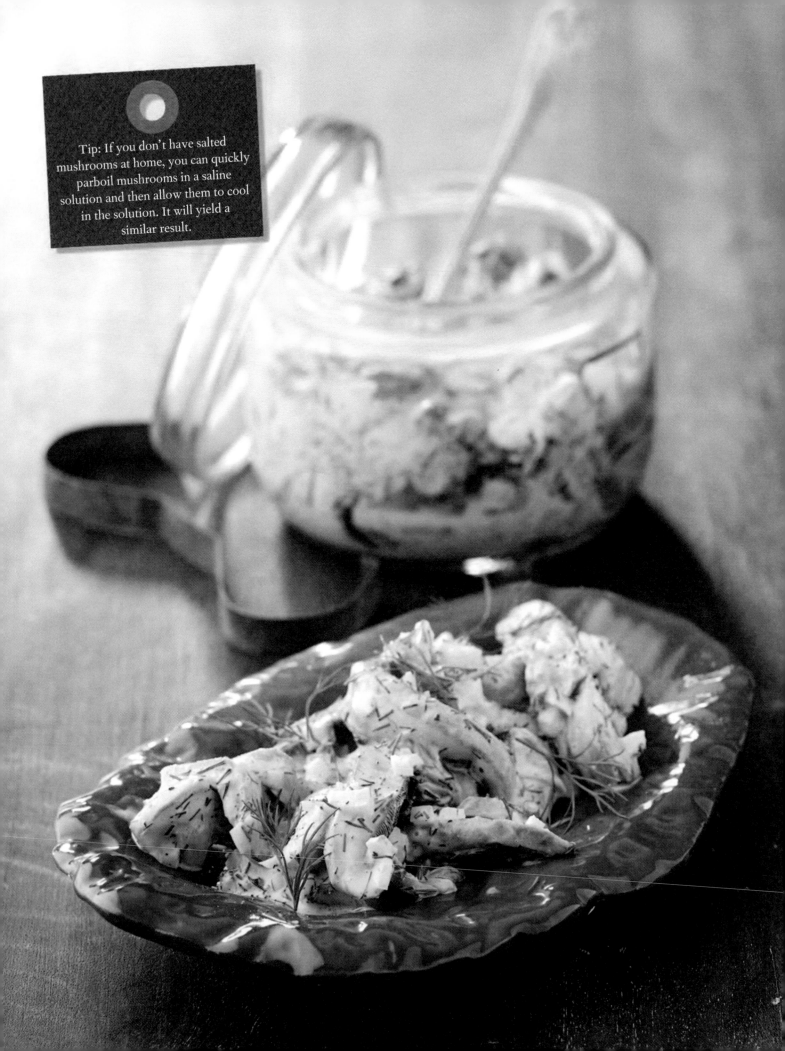

Tip: If you don't have salted mushrooms at home, you can quickly parboil mushrooms in a saline solution and then allow them to cool in the solution. It will yield a similar result.

Finnish Russian mushroom salad

Russians and Finns are experts in edible and non-edible mushrooms. You can actually eat parboiled and thoroughly soaked red hot milk caps! Not to mention bearded milk caps, northern bearded milk caps, ugly bearded milk caps, and pickle milk caps. After salting and soaking, even the most bitter milk cap can be used to make a traditional Finnish mushroom dish. I don't know much about milk caps, so I tend to use wood (or scaly) hedgehogs instead.

Salted mushrooms tend to last until the next mushroom season. Layer parboiled mushrooms with coarse salt in a jar, or a pot. Always begin and end with salt. Use a handful of salt for each mushroom layer. Perhaps $4/5$ cup (250 g) of salt for 34 oz (1 liter) of parboiled mushrooms. Try adding a tablespoon of whole white pepper, and perhaps some dill and garlic.

Traditionally, a few oak or black currant leaves are added before a weight is placed on top. I use a plastic bag filled with water. It is easier than trying to find little plates that will fit into the pot. Store in a cool place. After a few days, enough liquid will have seeped out from the mushrooms to cover them. Otherwise, you can press lightly on top of the plate. If you still don't have enough liquid to cover the mushrooms, just boil some salted water and add it. Once the mushrooms are covered with the saline solution, they will last for a few months without going rancid.

When it is time to use the mushrooms, thoroughly soak them for a few hours, and they will be like new. If they taste very salty, you may need to soak overnight.

17 oz (½ liter) soaked salted mushrooms
1 yellow onion, finely chopped
1 bunch chopped dill (at least)
1 jar crème fraiche (sour cream or smetana)
Pepper, if you wish

Cut the mushrooms as if you were making pickled herring.
   Mix with the remaining ingredients. Taste and adjust flavor if you need to.
   Store in a cool place for a few hours so that the flavors settle.

Guests that are unfamiliar with this dish often mistake it for herring! If you make this salad recipe for four people, you'll get about 3 grams of carbohydrates per person. The fat-burning quotient is 1.5.

Waldorf salad

See photo on page 48.

The Waldorf salad is a crispy blend of celery, apple, and walnuts with a creamy mayo dressing. It is a refreshing addition to fatty and smoked food.

1 bunch tender celery stalks
1 tart apple
$2/5$ cup (60 g) walnuts
$4/5$ cup (200 g) mayo dressing (see recipe on page 155)

Mix the ingredients for the dressing. Taste and adjust if needed. Stir the finely chopped celery into the dressing, then cut the apple into thin sticks, about the size of matches. Add walnuts and store salad in a cool place before serving it.

The carbohydrate value of this salad will vary depending on how much apple you add. 3.5 oz (1 hg) of apples will provide about 13 grams of carbohydrates! The celery and the mayo dressing are almost carbohydrate-free. If you are economical with the apple, and generous with the dressing, the fat-burning quotient will be about 3.

"Our entire humanity would have poor health if vegetables tasted as good as bacon."
/ SSS

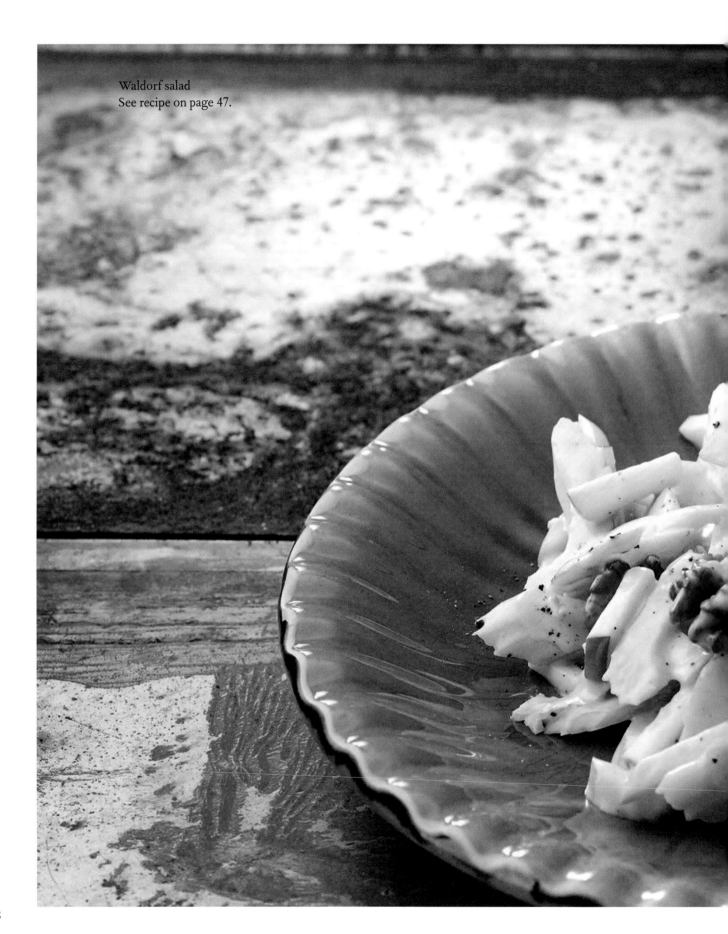

Waldorf salad
See recipe on page 47.

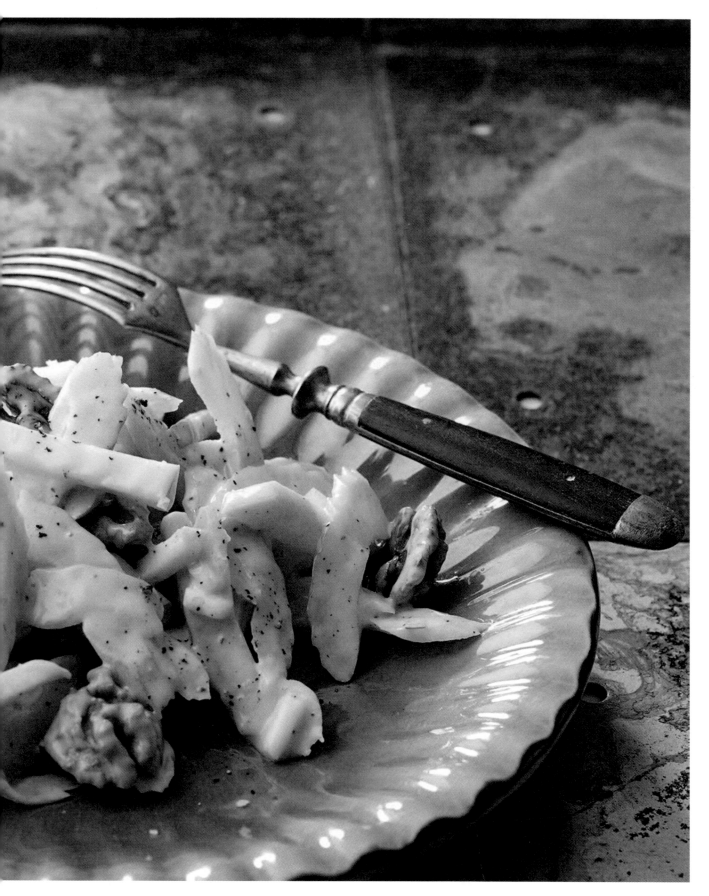

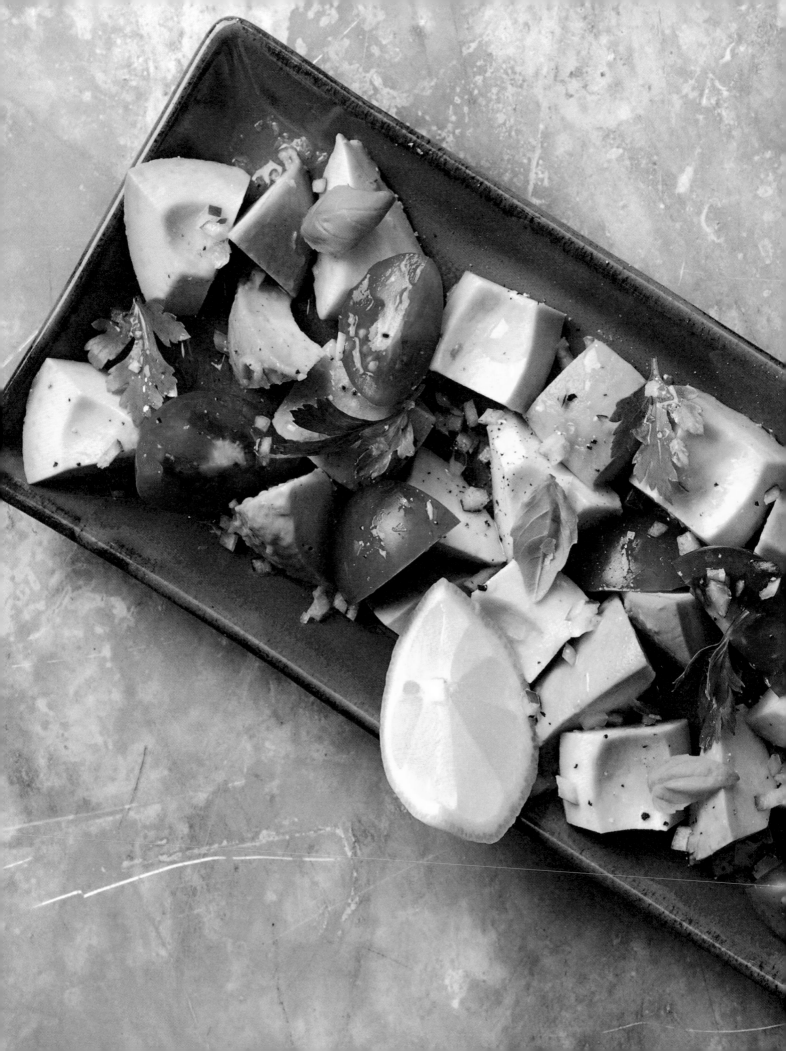

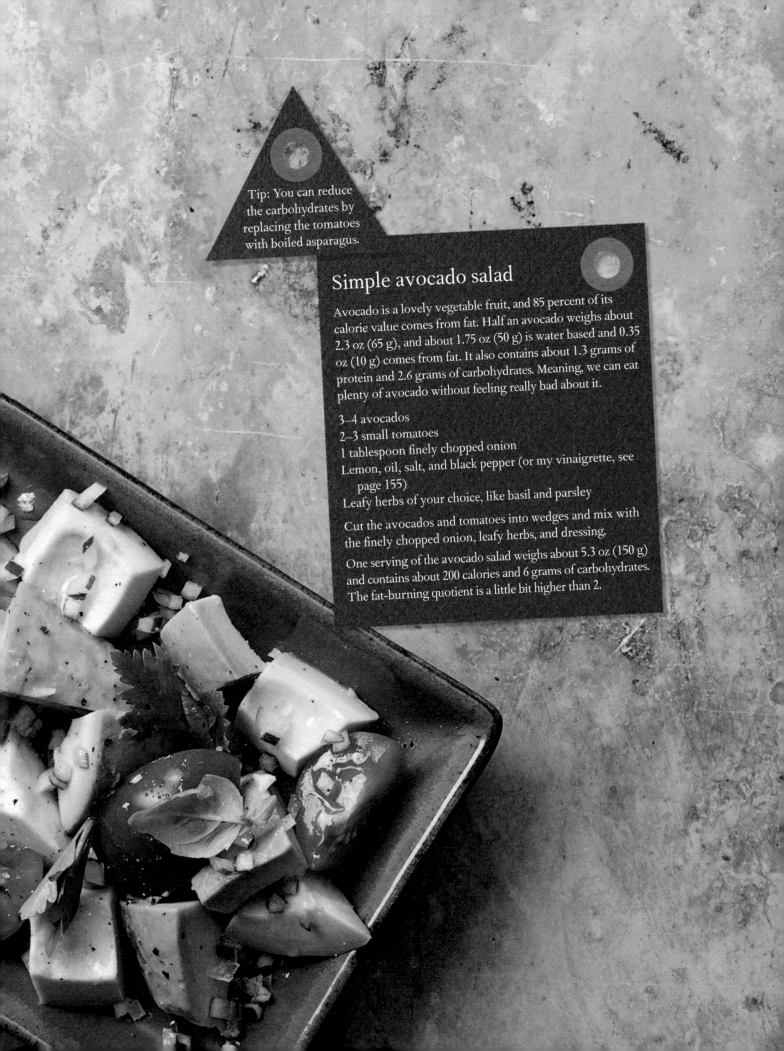

Tip: You can reduce the carbohydrates by replacing the tomatoes with boiled asparagus.

Simple avocado salad

Avocado is a lovely vegetable fruit, and 85 percent of its calorie value comes from fat. Half an avocado weighs about 2.3 oz (65 g), and about 1.75 oz (50 g) is water based and 0.35 oz (10 g) comes from fat. It also contains about 1.3 grams of protein and 2.6 grams of carbohydrates. Meaning, we can eat plenty of avocado without feeling really bad about it.

3–4 avocados
2–3 small tomatoes
1 tablespoon finely chopped onion
Lemon, oil, salt, and black pepper (or my vinaigrette, see page 155)
Leafy herbs of your choice, like basil and parsley

Cut the avocados and tomatoes into wedges and mix with the finely chopped onion, leafy herbs, and dressing.

One serving of the avocado salad weighs about 5.3 oz (150 g) and contains about 200 calories and 6 grams of carbohydrates. The fat-burning quotient is a little bit higher than 2.

Omelet with creamed mushrooms

I love to go mushroom picking and could eat mushrooms all year round. Mushrooms go well with any animal-based food. A mushroom cream stew is absolutely delectable in an omelet. Here is an old, classic recipe where you'll need to use the egg shells for measurement.

For the omelet:

3 eggs

3 eggshell halves of cream

Half an eggshell of mayonnaise

1 teaspoon *sambal oelek*

Salt and black pepper

For the mushroom filling:

34 oz (1 liter) fresh mushrooms

½ finely chopped yellow onion

1 crushed garlic clove (optional)

Butter to sauté the mushrooms

Cream or crème fraiche

Salt and pepper

Whisk together the ingredients for the omelet batter and allow to stand.

Begin by steaming the mushrooms over low heat in a pot. Once the liquid has evaporated, sauté the mushrooms in butter with the finely chopped onion. Add spices according to your own preference and taste.

Pour cream or crème fraiche over the mushrooms until they are covered and boil down to creamed mushrooms.

Now it's time to sauté the omelet. Once it looks the way you want it, you'll put the stew on one half of the omelet, and fold the other half over. I usually fold it as I slide the omelet onto a plate. With time, practice will ease this process. The seam of the filled omelet should preferably end up on the underside, but I find that to be a bit advanced.

This omelet is enough for two people. Each serving contains about 600 calories and 6 grams of carbohydrates. The fat-burning quotient is 3.

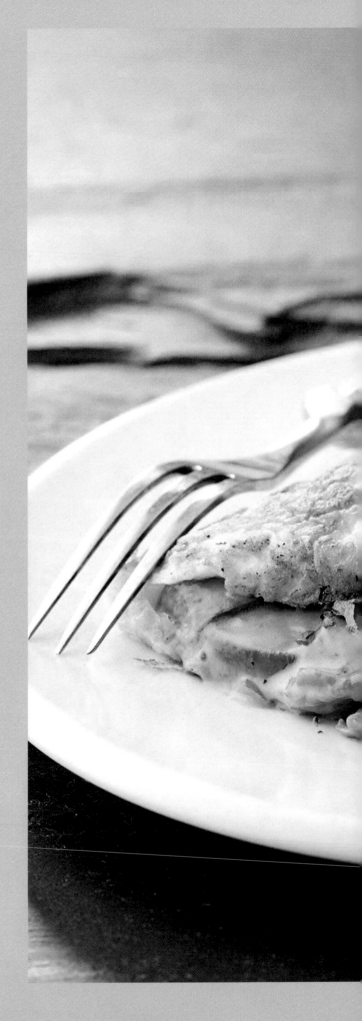

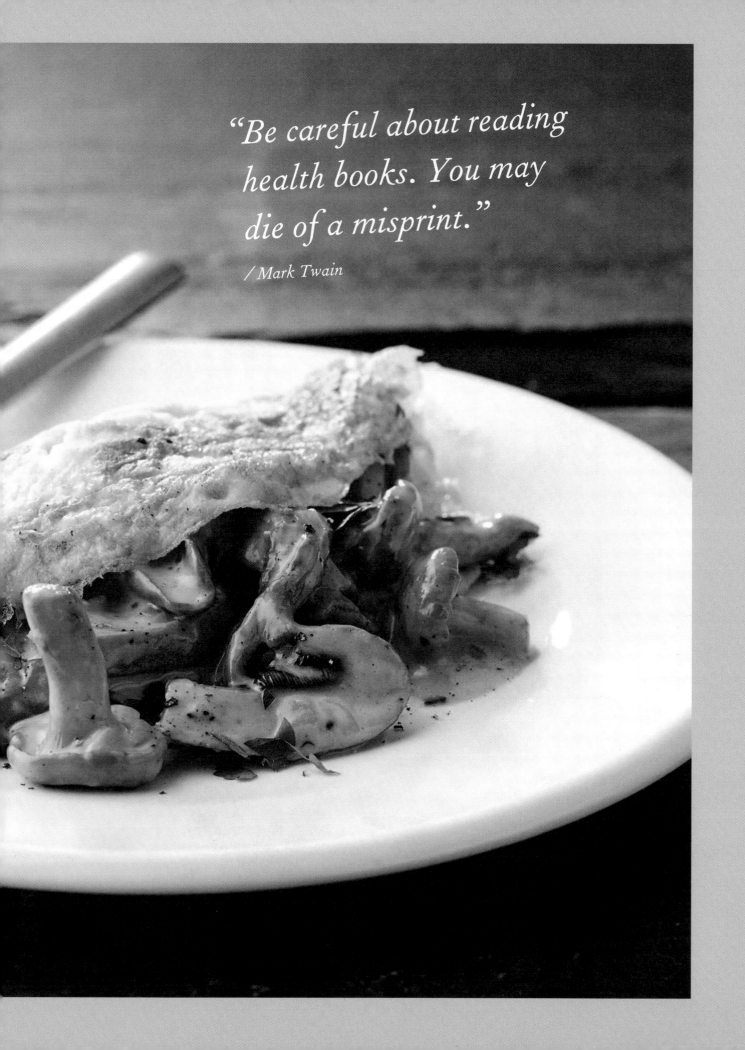

"*Be careful about reading health books. You may die of a misprint.*"

/ Mark Twain

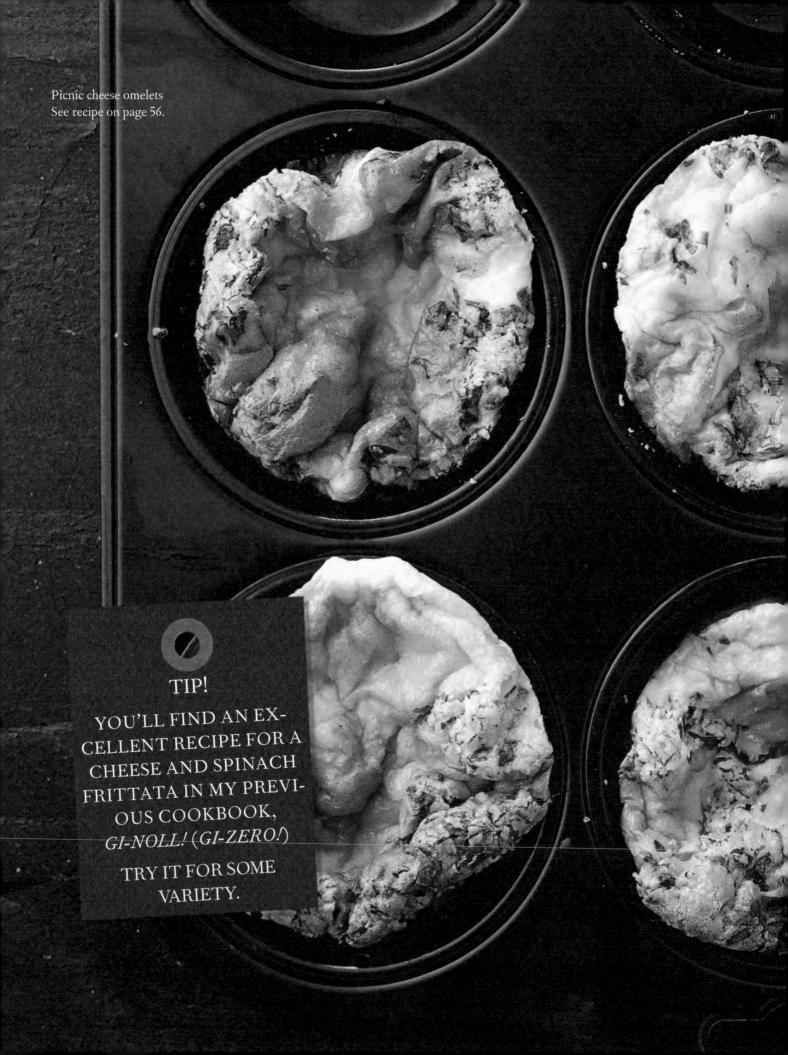

Picnic cheese omelets
See recipe on page 56.

TIP!
YOU'LL FIND AN EX-
CELLENT RECIPE FOR A
CHEESE AND SPINACH
FRITTATA IN MY PREVI-
OUS COOKBOOK,
GI-NOLL! (GI-ZERO!)

TRY IT FOR SOME
VARIETY.

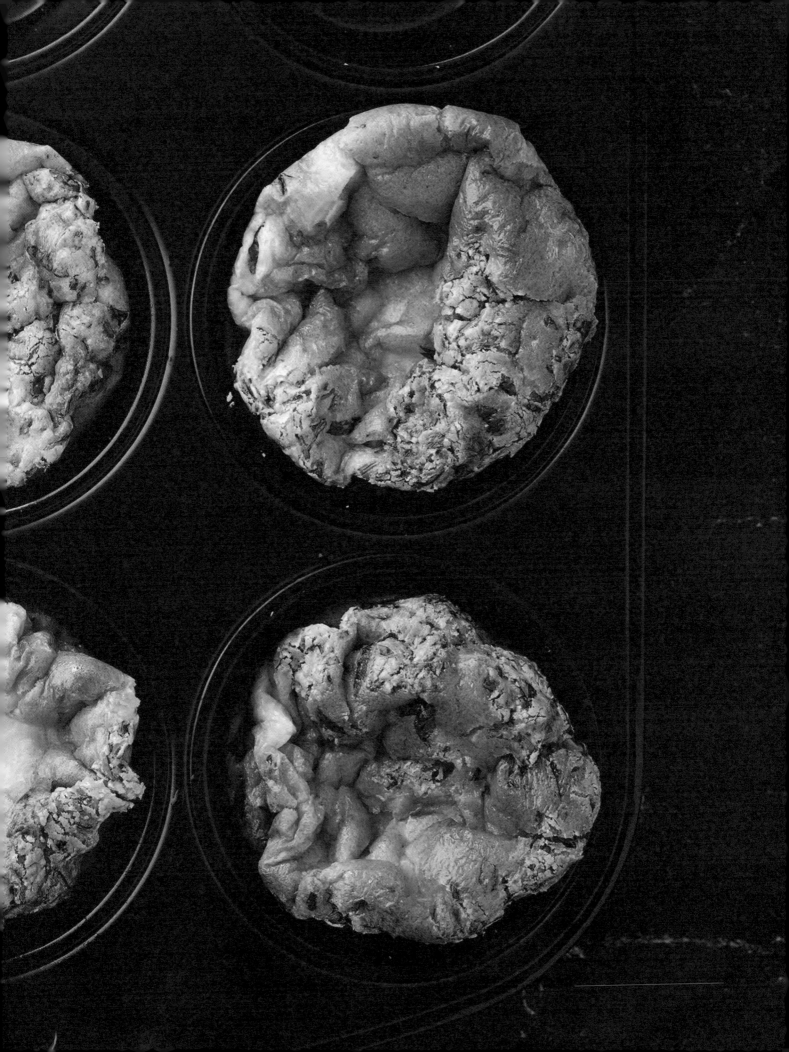

Picnic cheese omelets

See photo on page 54.

Cheese omelets are perfect little picnic treats. Grate some leftover cheese, mix with plenty of eggs, spice with black pepper, and bake in the oven. That's the basic recipe. I like to add a little bit of cream, but that's optional. Naturally, you can add more spices and flavors if you'd like, but green herbs, or something meat-based, such as bacon, sautéed chicken, or smoked fish, make a nice addition. If you bake the omelets in a muffin pan (the Teflon kind), you'll get perfect bite-size pieces for the picnic.

You'll need the following for a big pan:

10 eggs

1⅓ –1¾ cups (300–400 g) grated cheese, preferably several varieties

⅘ cup (200 ml) heavy whipping cream

Leafy herb spices of your choice

Pepper

Finely chopped chicken, or smoked salmon, or mackerel, or crispy bacon

Combine the ingredients and fill the (buttered) muffin pans with the batter. Bake in a fairly warm oven until the omelets have a nice golden-brown color. It takes about 20 minutes.

A small omelet is about 230 calories and contains about 1 gram of carbohydrates.

The fat-burning quotient is 1.25. If you eat your mini omelet with a tablespoon of butter, you'll get another 100 calories, and the fat-burning quotient will increase to about 2.0.

Filled omelet

An omelet with filling is ideal for the LCHF diet. Here is a simple and quick variation that I made the other day by throwing together ingredients I happened to have at home. I mixed everything together in the pan. It's always an advantage not to whisk the omelet batter too much.

½ package of bacon

1 tablespoon cooking fat

1 tablespoon finely chopped onion

2–3 eggs

⅖ cup (100 g) heavy whipping cream

⅖ cup (100 g) crayfish tails in solution

⅘ cup (200 g) grated flavorful cheese

Black pepper

Cut the bacon into pieces directly into a Teflon pan and sauté lightly in cooking fat. Spread onion on top and cook until shiny. Crack the eggs into the pan. Add the cream and two tablespoons of the crayfish solution. Mix with a spatula until everything is thoroughly blended. You shouldn't touch the batter again; the omelet should just barely stick together.

While the omelet is cooking over medium heat, grate about ⅘ cup (200 g) of any flavorful cheese of your choice; I recommend Västerbotten cheese. Spread the cheese over the omelet and allow it to melt. Once the top of the omelet begins to solidify, top it off with about ⅖ cup (100 g) of crayfish tails. Grind some fresh black pepper over it. Salt isn't necessary. The shrimp, solution, cheese, and bacon have enough salt to flavor the omelet. Now it's time to serve the meal.

Loosen the omelet around the edges and make sure that it has a nice color underneath. Allow it to glide halfway onto a warm plate. Fold over the other half on top. Eat and enjoy!

This omelet is a great complete meal for someone who's hungry, or it could be divided into a lighter meal for two people. The entire omelet (made with 2 eggs) contains about 1,100 calories, 59 grams of protein, 98 grams of fat, and 7 grams of carbohydrates. The fat-burning quotient is 1.5. This omelet is packed with nutrients and contains plenty of vitamins and minerals. It provides three days' worth of saturated fat and almost two days' worth of cholesterol. A meal like this builds up your cell walls, stimulates sex hormones, and strengthens your immune system.

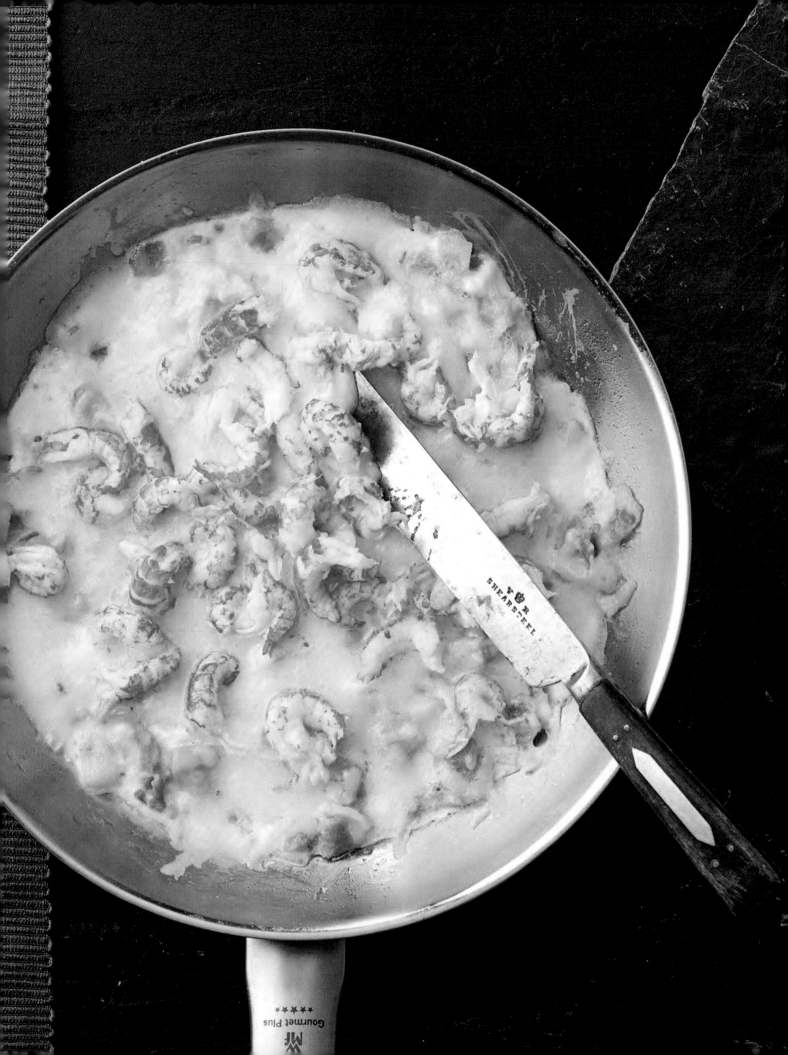

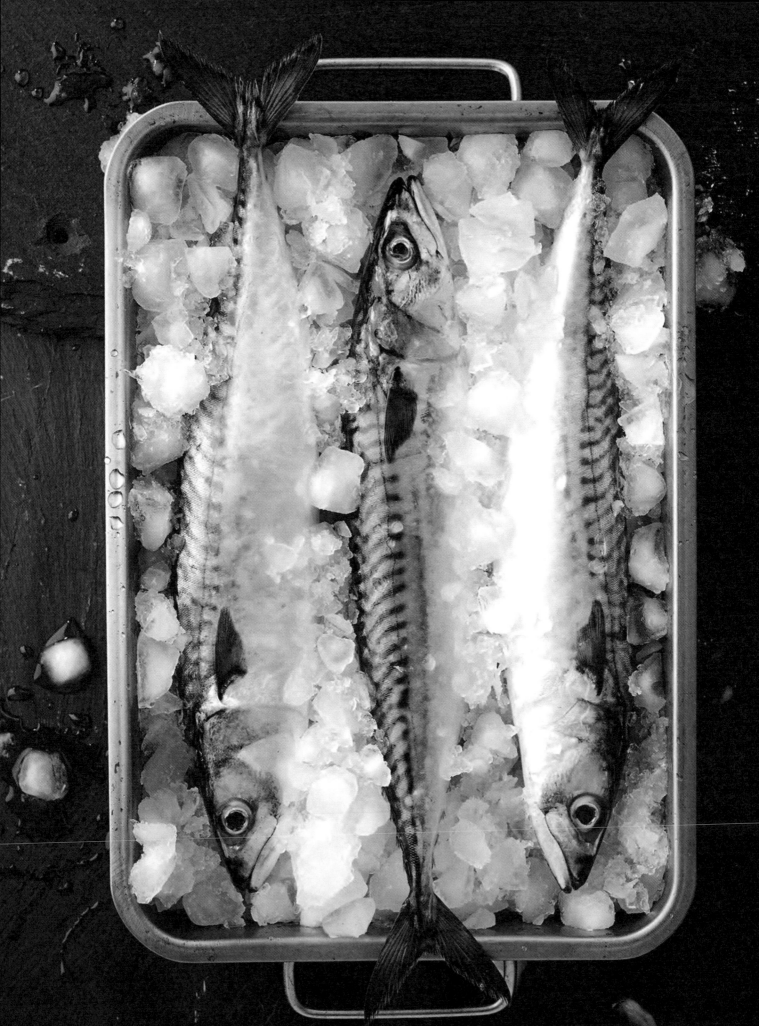

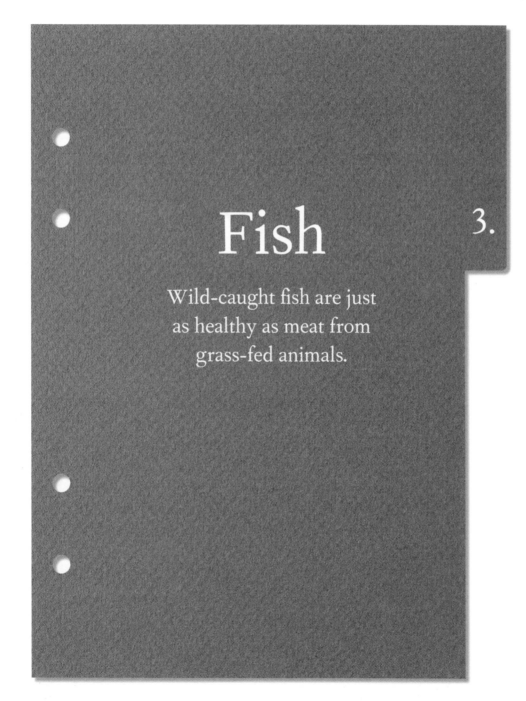

Fish

3.

Wild-caught fish are just
as healthy as meat from
grass-fed animals.

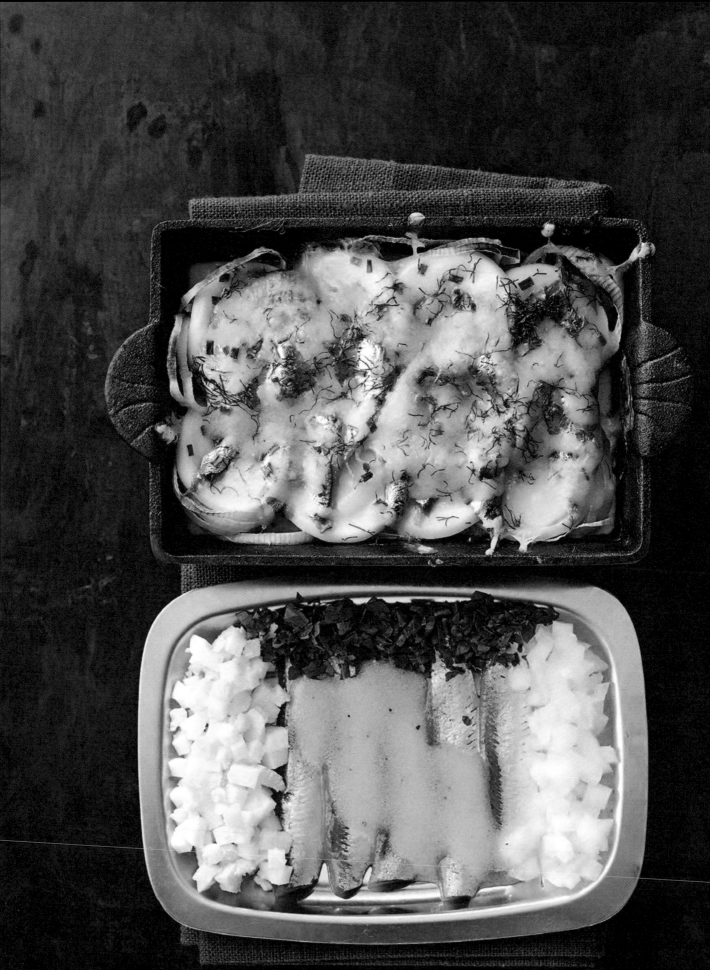

Two small anchovy dishes

Anchovies are delicious, especially during the summer. They provide us with our necessary salt intake and are often served with eggs, which are very healthy for us. The only issue is that anchovies contain a lot of carbohydrates. Some canned anchovy brands are the worst, with about 14 grams of carbohydrates per 3.5 oz (1 hg). Use the fillets, but avoid the sugar-rich solution that they come in.

About thirty years ago, we weren't afraid of fat. We managed to maintain a healthy weight anyway, and therefore Arla Foods was able to print recipes like the following:

Egg and anchovy box

A little bit of shredded leek
4 hardboiled eggs
1 can anchovies, about 4.4 oz (125 g)
Dill or chives
⅖–⅘ cup (100–200 ml) heavy whipping cream, let's use ⅘ cup (200 ml)!
Grated cheese, as high in fat as possible

Shred the leek and place it in a buttered pan.

Slice the eggs and spread them over the leek. Drain the anchovy fillets and place them on top. Top off with finely cut dill or chives.

Lastly, pour the cream and spread the grated cheese on top.

Bake in the oven at 425–450°F (225–250°C) for about 10 minutes.

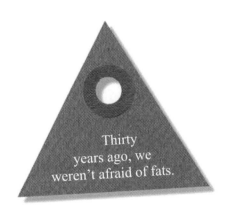

Thirty years ago, we weren't afraid of fats.

Summer dish with anchovies and eggs

Here is a golden recipe from the book *GI-Noll!* (*GI-Zero!*). It is excellent when the summer heat is pressing outside. That's when we need salt, and the anchovies will take care of that. Together with chopped eggs, onion, and dressing, it's a delicious summer meal when we crave something a little bit lighter.

Anchovy fillets, about 5 per serving
2 hardboiled eggs per person
Yellow onion or shredded leek
Parsley
Vinegar dressing (see page 155)

Elegantly spread the anchovy fillets in the center of a plate.

Chop the remaining ingredients and spread them around the fillets. Drizzle with vinegar dressing and store in a cool place for 30 minutes.

Recipes based on eggs and carbohydrates contain about 8 grams of carbohydrates per serving. We're talking about appetizers. Normally, we add butter or cream, and therefore achieve a better fat-burning quotient, around 1.5. If that's too many carbohydrates for you, skip some of the fillets and eat more eggs instead.

Horseradish-cured Atlantic herring
See recipe on page 64.

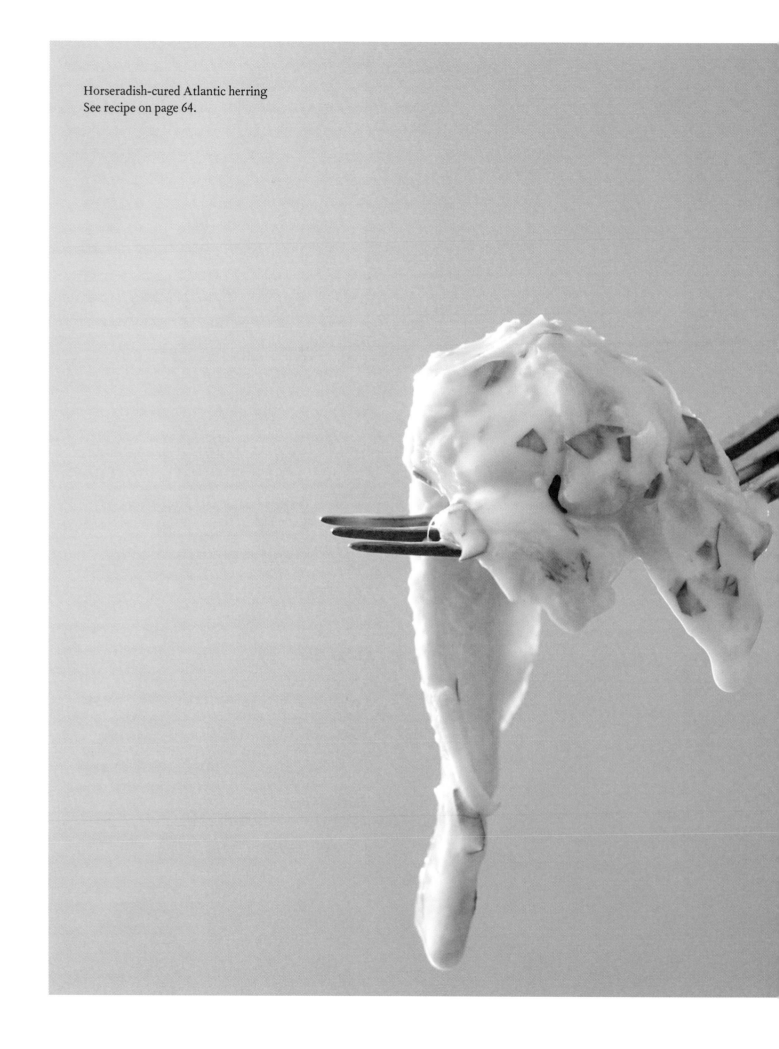

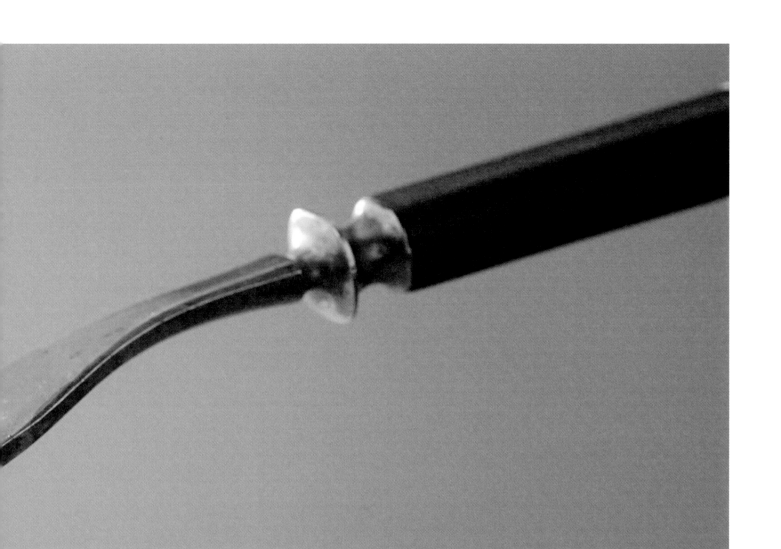

"The benefit of this Atlantic herring is that there is no added sugar in the solution."

Horseradish-cured Atlantic herring

See recipe photo on page 62.

In one magazine, I noticed a recipe for Ulla Winbladh's Atlantic herring. It was probably intended as a Christmas dish, but it is even better during the summer. The benefit of this Atlantic herring is that there is no added sugar in the solution.

I have made many different variations of this dish, but the original recipe is just fine. You should prepare this meal at least a day ahead, because you'll need to cure the herring in two rounds: First, in a vinegar solution, and later, in horseradish sauce. Therefore, you may as well make a big batch while you are at it.

2.2 lbs (1 kg) cleaned Atlantic herring

For the vinegar solution:
At least 34 oz (1 liter) water
⅘ cup (200 ml) vinegar
2 tablespoons salt

For the horseradish sauce:
1⅓ cups (300 g) mayonnaise
1⅓ cups (300 g) crème fraiche
1 tablespoon Dijon mustard
⅖ cup (13 g) chopped parsley
4–5 tablespoons freshly grated horseradish
1–2 teaspoons Worcestershire sauce
White pepper
Salt
(The original recipe calls for sugar, but we will skip it.)

Day 1:
Mix the ingredients for the solution. Put the boneless herring into the solution and store in the fridge overnight.

Day 2:
Mix the horseradish sauce, taste, and make any adjustments if needed. I like mine pretty spicy.

Drain the fillets from the solution before you put them in the horseradish sauce. If you do this in the morning, the herring will be ready to eat by the evening

The horseradish herring is fatty and fairly low in carbohydrates. It contains healthy fats and plenty of vitamin B12, vitamin D, and vitamin E. Most of the carbohydrates in this meal come from the crème fraiche. Count on about 3–4 grams per serving. If you eat the sauce, the fat-burning quotient will exceed 2.

Rikard's salmon gratin

I have a very nice letter exchange going with some of the people that read my health books. I receive everything from success stories to questions. Every once in a while, I'll even get a recipe, like this one from Rikard in Gotheburg, Sweden. It has all the qualities I look for in a recipe: It's simple to make, delicious to eat, and super-healthy for the body.

2 salmon fillets, 4.4–5.3 oz (125–150 g) each, preferably with the skin for extra flavor
½ broccoli head, divided into little florets and lightly parboiled
3.5 oz (100 g) fresh mushrooms, cut into halves
3.5 oz (100 g) peeled shrimp
1 piece of mozzarella, thinly sliced

For the sauce:
3.5–4.4 oz (100–125 g) crème fraiche
3.5–4.4 oz (100–125 g) mayonnaise
1–2 egg yolks
1 tablespoon tomato purée
A little bit of fresh lemon juice, or perhaps some white wine
Plenty of basil

Place the salmon fillets next to each other in a small oven-proof dish.

Spread mushrooms and broccoli around the fillets, shrimp in the middle, and mozzarella on top.

Mix the ingredients for the sauce and cover the gratin.

Bake in the oven at 350°F (175°C), about 24–30 minutes.

This dish is healthy and fairly rich. One serving contains over 1,000 calories, 6–8 grams of carbohydrates, and the fat-burning quotient is about 1.5.

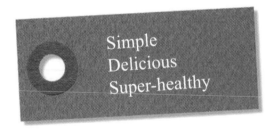

Simple
Delicious
Super-healthy

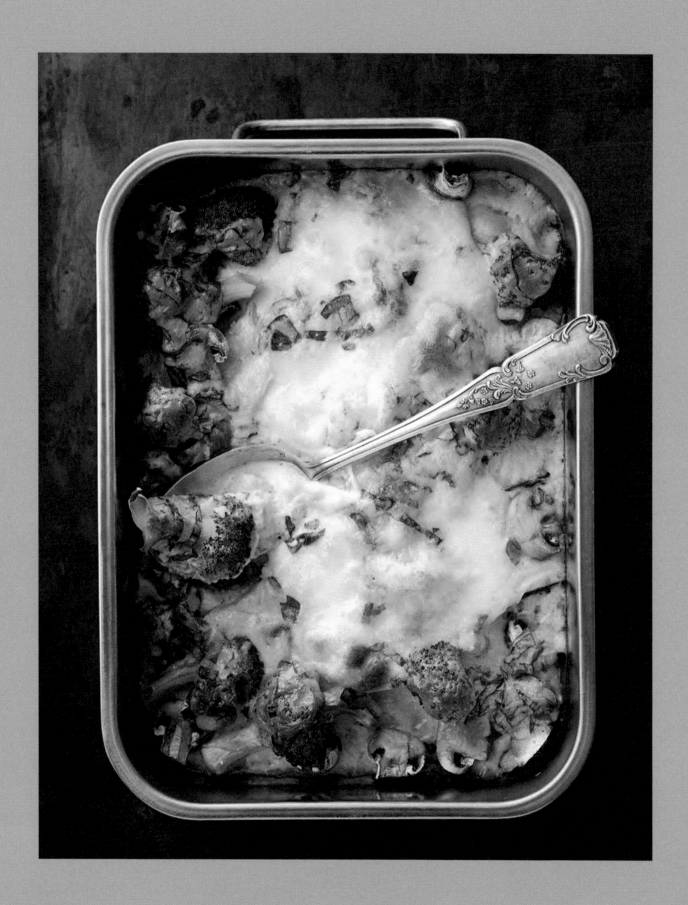

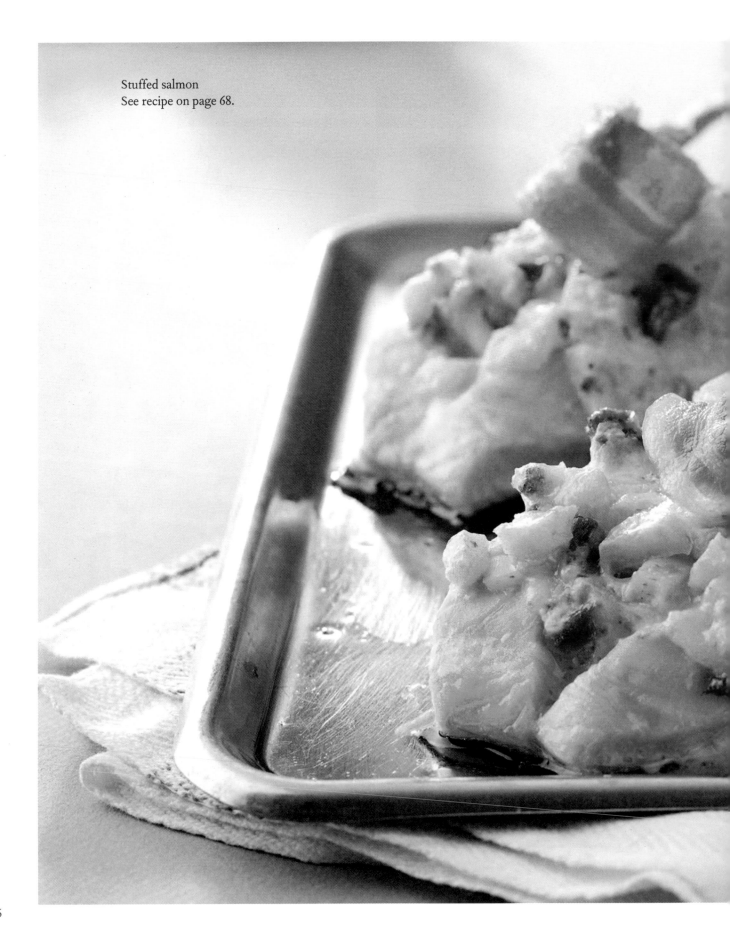

Stuffed salmon
See recipe on page 68.

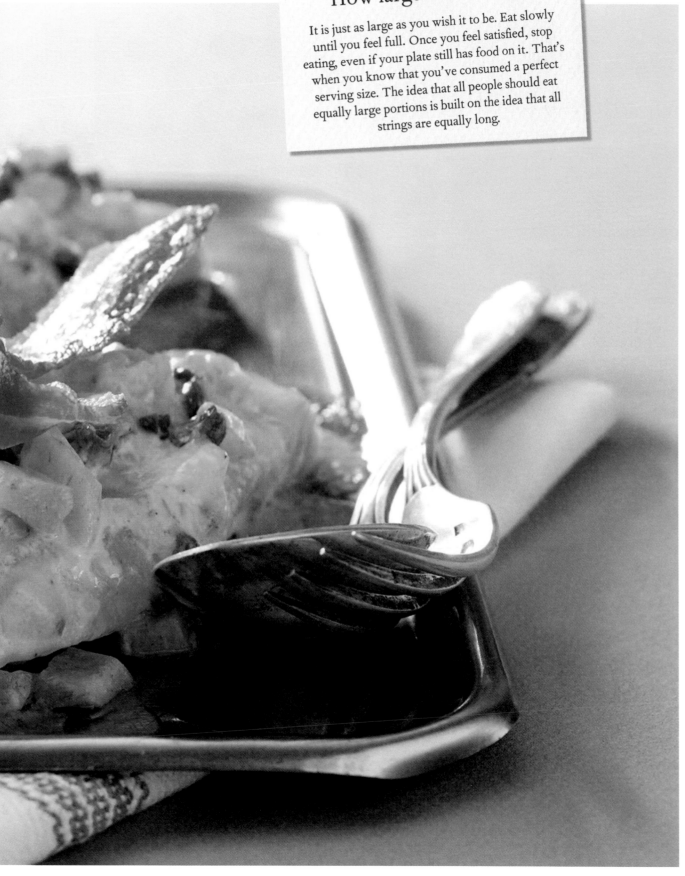

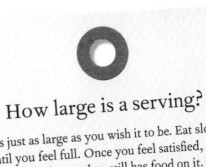

How large is a serving?

It is just as large as you wish it to be. Eat slowly until you feel full. Once you feel satisfied, stop eating, even if your plate still has food on it. That's when you know that you've consumed a perfect serving size. The idea that all people should eat equally large portions is built on the idea that all strings are equally long.

> *"Fishing is the only philosophical activity that fills you up."*
> /Norwegian proverb

Stuffed salmon

See photo on page 66.

4 salmon fillets with skin

Filling:
⅖ cup (100 g) crème fraiche
½ can of artichoke bottoms, finely chopped
⅖ cup (100 g) grated Västerbotten cheese, or any other flavorful cheese
4 finely chopped sundried tomatoes (FYI: rich in carbohydrates!)
Salt and pepper

For the garnish:
4 slices of crispy bacon

Place the bacon slices on a baking sheet and dry in the oven at 350°F (175°C).

Mix the ingredients for the filling. Taste and add spices accordingly.

Use a knife to make deep cuts in the salmon fillets and press the filling into the crevices. Sauté the salmon at 350°F (175°C) for about 20 minutes.

Cut bacon strips over the salmon as decoration (the original recipe suggests oven-dried prosciutto, but I prefer bacon).

Try serving this salmon with a refreshing green salad (see page 39).

A filled salmon fillet contains about 700 calories and 6 grams of carbohydrates. The fat-burning quotient is 1. Half of the carbohydrates in this dish come from the tiny portion of sundried tomatoes. You can replace them with pesto if you want a low-carbohydrate alternative.

Cognac gravlax

I recommend using the fillets from a large salmon that weighs about 8.8 pounds (4 kg) or more. That will leave you with about 4.4 pounds (2 kg) of bone-free fillets, which is good for twenty appetizers or ten main courses. Cut the fillets and use the insides of both fillets (if you are afraid of parasites, freeze the salmon before and after curing it for 4–5 days). Gravlax will last about ten days in the fridge, but a few months if you keep it in the freezer.

For the spice blend:
1 bunch dill (fresh)
⅖ cup (100 g) sugar
⅘ cup (200 g) salt
15 white peppercorns
10 juniper berries
4 tablespoons cognac

Crush white pepper and juniper berries in a mortar, add sugar and salt, and rub generously over the salmon fillets.

Add the chopped dill and turn the fillets towards each other, with the skin side outwards. Transfer them to a plastic bag and fill it with the cognac. Seal the bag and store the salmon in the fridge.

Turn the bag at least once a day, and leave the salmon in there for about three days.

This food is very healthy and versatile. My good friend Lars-Evert, who created this recipe, uses this salmon as an appetizer, main course, and for the smorgasbord. Only the sides will vary. As an appetizer, you can serve this salmon with an egg scramble (see recipe on page 52), and a good, sugar-free mustard. As a main course, I tend to serve this with a delicious Waldorf salad (see page 41), 2 boiled eggs, and French mustard. The salmon contains almost no carbohydrates, and there is 1 carbohydrate in the eggs. You can add the Waldorf salad if you won't feel bad about it.

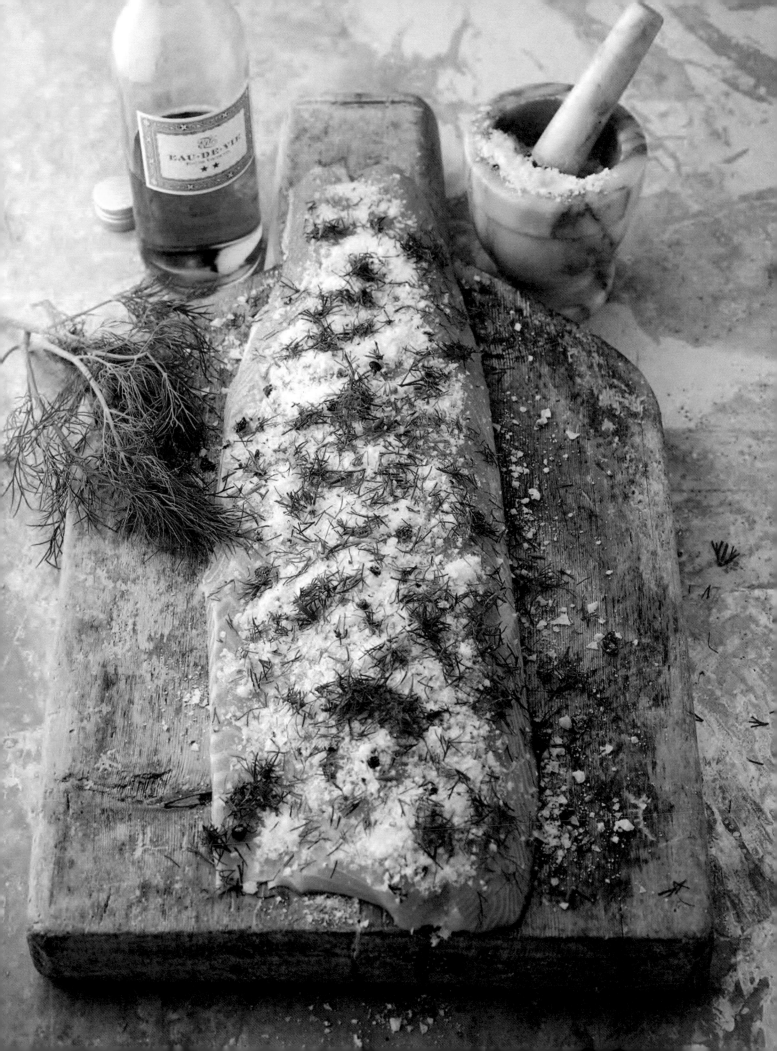

Fish à la Florentine

Turbot, Torbay sole, common sole, brill, or zander
 (you can use almost any type of white fish fillets)
 Use whole fish; about 2.2–3.8 lbs (1–1¾ kg) for 4 portions
1.3 lbs (600 g) spinach
10 cocktail tomatoes
(4 lemon wedges)

Clean and fillet the fish. Place the fillets in cold, salted water for 5–10 minutes. Boil the remaining parts of the fish to make a broth. You can use fish broth cubes if you can't find whole fish.

 Parboil the spinach in lightly salted water for a few minutes. Transfer to a colander and allow the water to drain off (or use frozen, chopped spinach).

 Sauté the spinach in plenty of butter and season lightly.

 Remove the fish fillets from the cold, salted water and allow any excess liquid to drain off. Spread the fillets in a fish pan, preferably with a grid. Strain the broth through a sieve over the fish until it is completely covered in the liquid. Cover with a lid and poach the fish for about 8–10 minutes.

 Strain the fish broth through a sieve and use it for the hollandaise sauce (see page 158).

 Keep the fish warm under the lid while you are cooking the sauce.

 Spread the sautéed spinach on a warm serving plate. Carefully lift out the fish from the grid (pan), allowing it to drain for a moment, then place it on top of the spinach. Spread the sauce over the fish.

 Garnish with the tomatoes. This elegant dish is excellent for lunch or dinner. One serving contains about 4–5 grams of carbohydrates and has a fat-burning quotient of about 1.

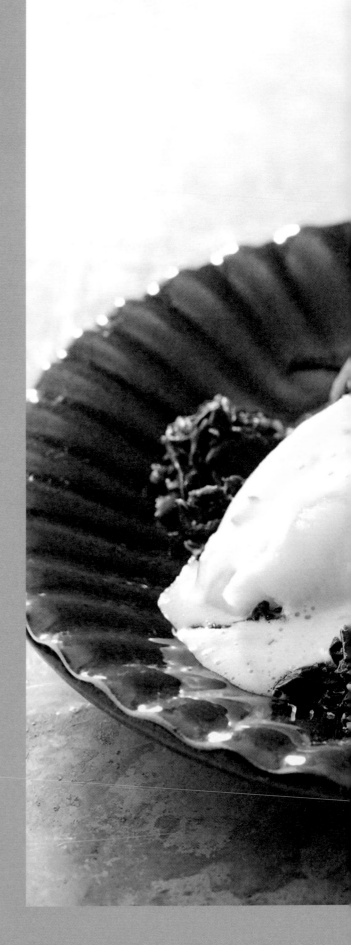

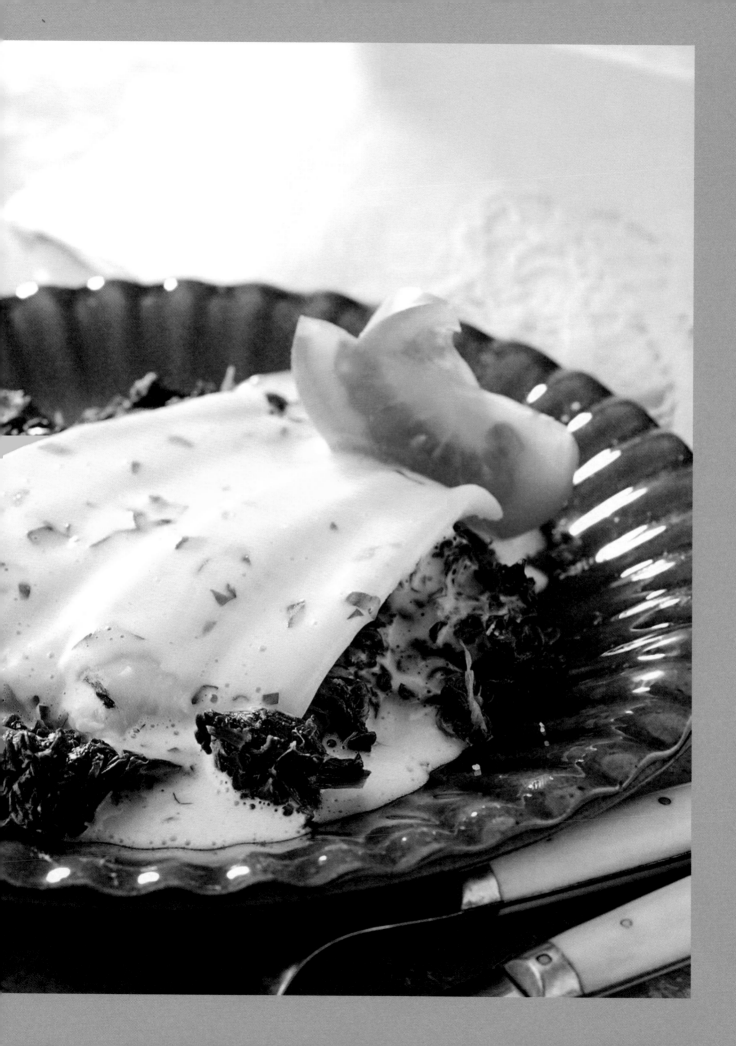

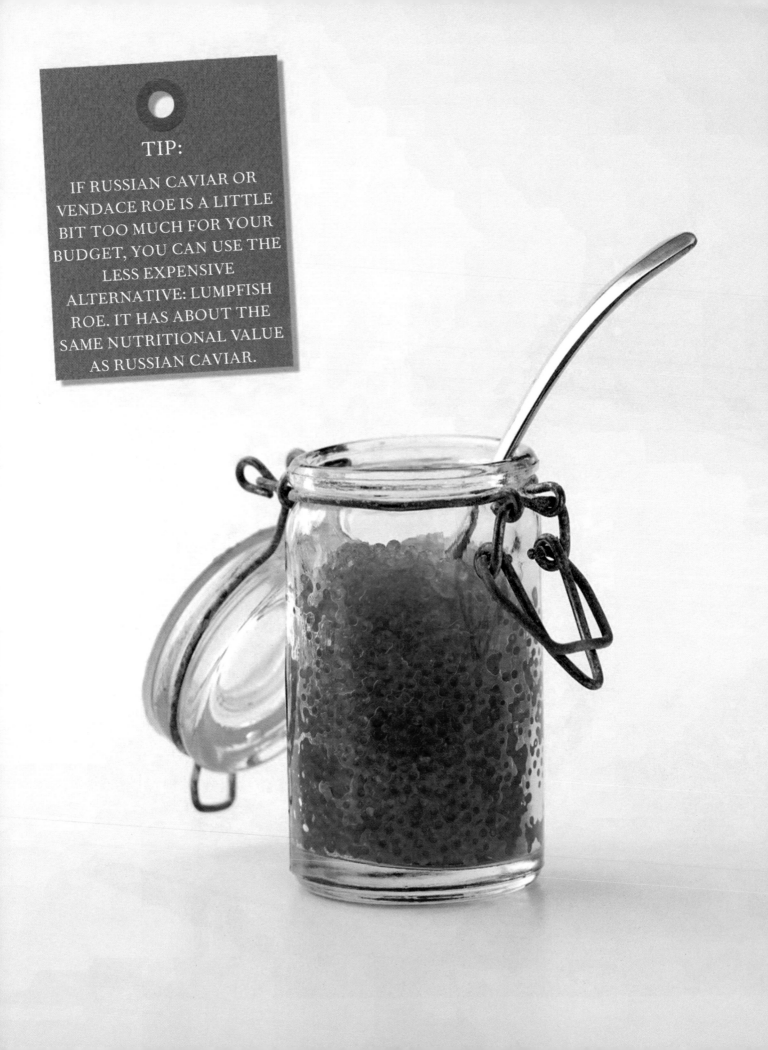

TIP:

IF RUSSIAN CAVIAR OR VENDACE ROE IS A LITTLE BIT TOO MUCH FOR YOUR BUDGET, YOU CAN USE THE LESS EXPENSIVE ALTERNATIVE: LUMPFISH ROE. IT HAS ABOUT THE SAME NUTRITIONAL VALUE AS RUSSIAN CAVIAR.

About caviar

There are many different types of caviar. If you buy it by the tube, the preferred kind to pick is smoked, or mildly smoked. Then you'll get a product that contains about 10–15 E percent carbohydrates and a good amount of fat. A tablespoon of smoked caviar contains about 2 grams of carbohydrates, about the same sugar value as in 3.5 oz (1 hg) of mayonnaise. The tube of smoked caviar has a fat-burning quotient of about 1.5.

An egg with a tablespoon of smoked caviar contains about 2.5 grams of carbohydrates and has a fat-burning quotient that is close to 1.0. Eat the egg with mayo if you want to raise the fat-burning quotient. One egg with one tablespoon of mayo contains about 0.7 grams of carbohydrates and has a fat-burning quotient of about 2.7.

The types of caviar that aren't smoked contain a fair amount of carbohydrates; half of the energy value may come from sugar. The fat burning quotient is often below 0.1. The unsmoked Slottskaviar brand is one of the better kinds, with barely 2 grams of carbohydrates per tablespoon and a fat-burning quotient at 0.13.

Real Russian caviar differs in nutritional value. A tablespoon of Russian caviar contains about 39 calories. About 40 percent of that energy value comes from protein. The fat value is pretty fair (53 E%), and the carbohydrate value is low. A tablespoon of Russian caviar contains about half a gram of carbohydrates. Because it is so rich in protein, the fat-burning quotient is only 0.5, but that is acceptable with food that you eat in small quantities.

If you want a higher protein value, vendace roe is a good choice. Seventy-eight percent of its energy value stems from protein, and it is low in fat and carbohydrates.

Low-carbohydrate Jansson temptation
See recipe on page 76.

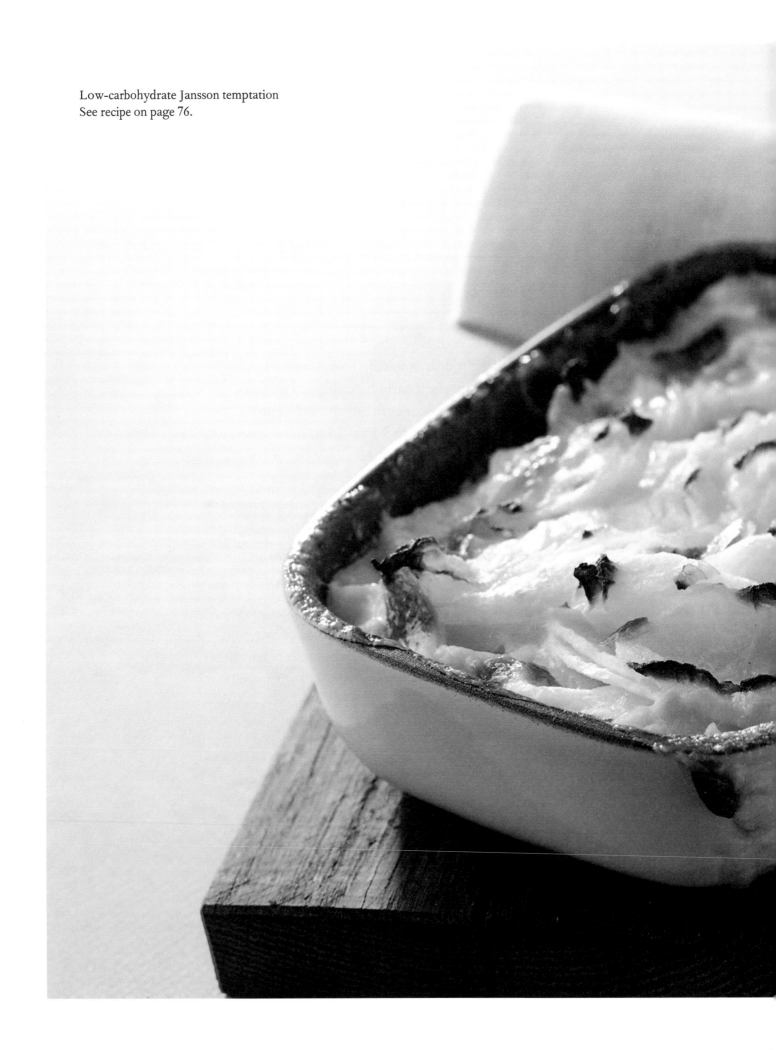

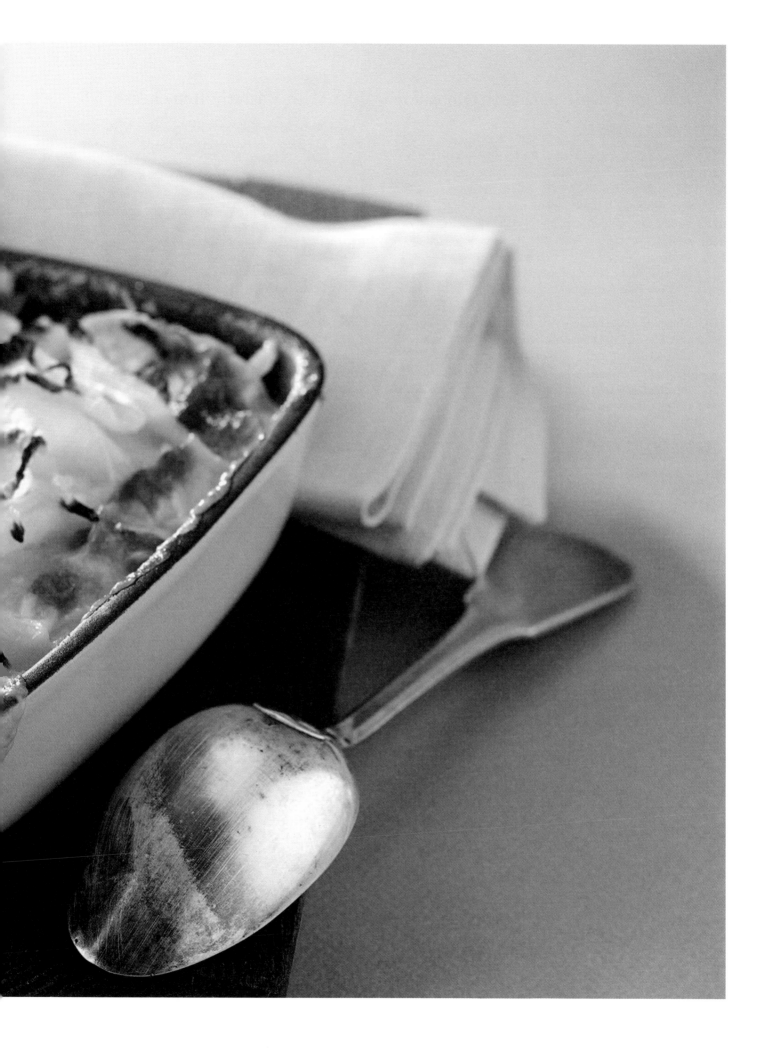

Low-carbohydrate Jansson temptation

See photo on page 74.

People are creatures of habit. We love to keep the foods we are used to eating, but we don't want to keep the foods that make us fat and sick. We want to try avoid eating carbohydrates. Is there a solution to this issue? Yes, there is. The best solution is to replace root vegetables that contain a lot of starch with root vegetables that contain hardly any starch. The only great alternative is daikon. It is related to the radish but has a much milder taste.

3.5 oz (100 g) contains 2.5 grams of carbohydrates and a whole lot of vitamin C. 3.5 oz (100 g) of boiled potatoes contain 18 grams of carbohydrates and barely anything else. The choice is simple. But what are we going to make with the daikon? From a flavor standpoint, Jansson's temptation is a clear winner. The daikon is so delicious in this dish that hardly anyone will notice that it isn't made the traditional way with potatoes.

A few large daikon roots
Yellow onion
Anchovies
Heavy whipping cream
Butter
Salt
White pepper
(Cheese)

Peel the daikon and slice thinly, then parboil for 15 minutes in salted water.

Drain the daikon from the water. Sauté a few chopped onions in butter. I usually add the daikon towards the end just to steam them off a bit more. Daikon tends to retain a lot of water.

Spread a layer of daikon and onion at the bottom of a pan. Spread anchovies on top. Drizzle with some of the anchovy liquid. Use one can for a small pan, and two cans for a large pan.

Cover with another layer of onion and daikon.

Dab some butter on top and pour heavy whipping cream over so that it barely covers the layers. If you want, you can add some grated cheese on top. I tend to skip the cheese.

Bake in the oven at 425°F (225°C) until the casserole has a nice color. It takes about 20 minutes.

One serving of this Jansson is 8.8 oz (250 g), contains just under 400 calories, and has about 10 grams of carbohydrates. The fat-burning quotient is higher than 2. This is a real diet dish. The equivalent portion of a traditional Jansson's temptation with potatoes would be under 300 calories, have about 30 grams of carbohydrates, and the fat-burning quotient would be under 0.4.

Fish with Västerbotten cheese

Västerbotten cheese is the Swedish equivalent of Parmesan cheese, and it replaces Parmesan in all the dishes. You can use Västerbotten cheese in any kind of oven-baked dishes. Try mixing some grated cheese with two licks of butter and place it on beef or fish. You can make a Västerbotten pesto by mixing together Västerbotten cheese, sundried tomatoes, and crème fraiche. The only thing you can't use Västerbotten cheese for is a sandwich!

In this recipe, we slice some Västerbotten cheese over the fish. Delicious with Arctic char!

Place the fish fillets in a buttered pan.
Season with salt and pepper.
Slice red onion (or leek) over the fish.
Cover with thinly sliced Västerbotten cheese, and last but not least, pour cream into the pan!
Bake in the oven at 400°F (200°C) until the fish has a nice color.

I've made this dish with freshly caught char, and it is absolutely delicious! Great with creamed spinach. The fish itself is pretty much carbohydrate-free, and the fat-burning quotient is about 1.1.

My creamed spinach (see page 145) adds about 2 grams of carbohydrates per serving that is 3.5 oz (1 hg) and brings up the fat-burning quotient to about 1.5.

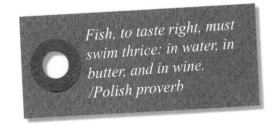

Fish, to taste right, must swim thrice: in water, in butter, and in wine.
/Polish proverb

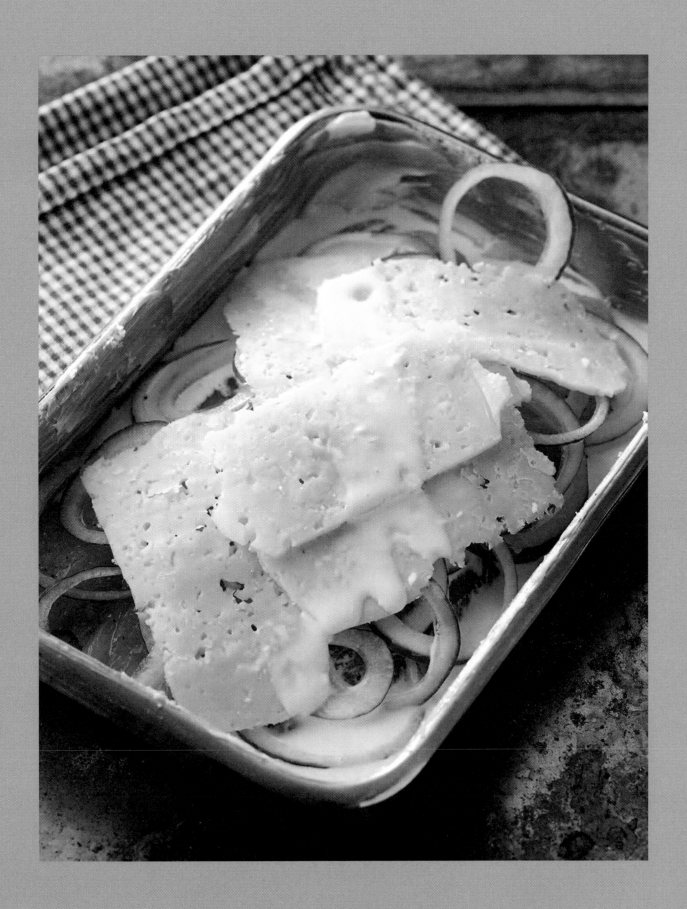

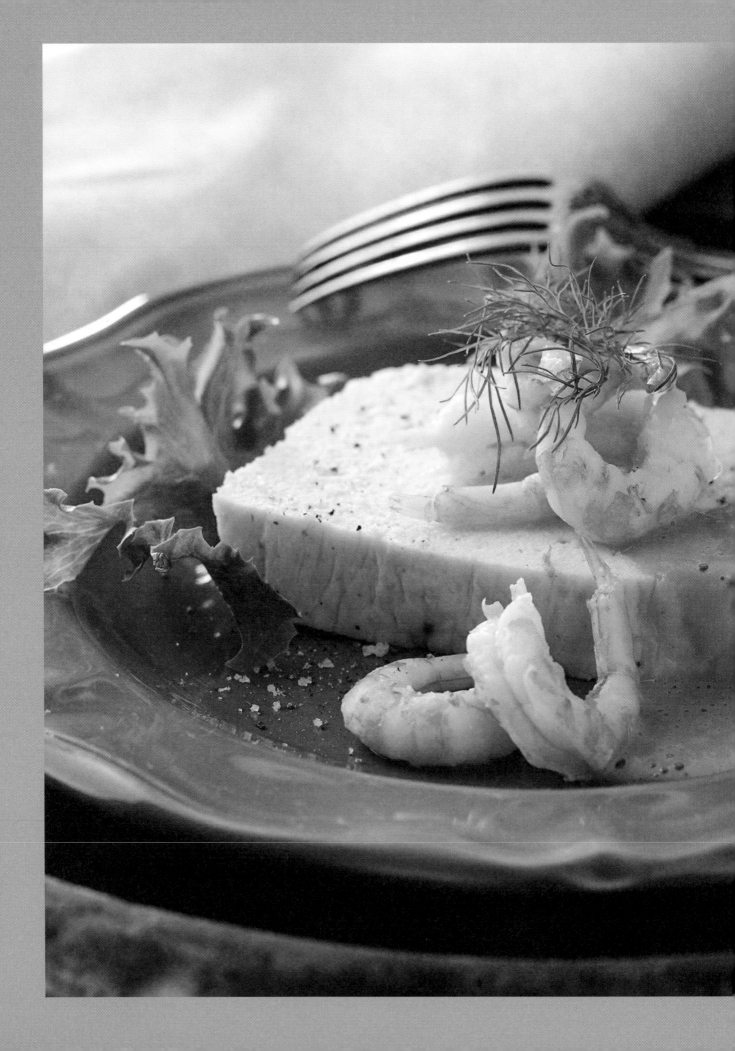

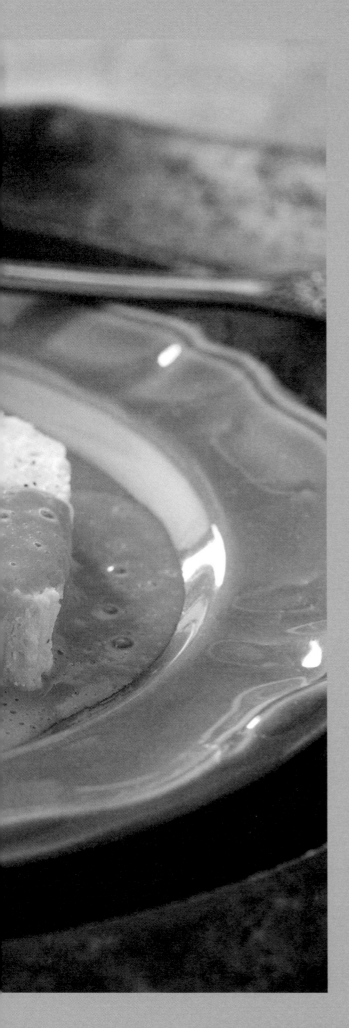

Elisabeth's pike and salmon mousse

We love all types of pike mousse, but I don't have time to go fishing too often. And I prefer to eat the fish freshly caught. We'll solve that issue by adding salmon to the pike to make it last longer.

10 oz (300 g) pike fillet
10 oz (300 g) salmon
6 eggs
2.5 cups (600 ml) heavy whipping cream
Spices, according to your own preference. We use salt, white pepper, a pinch of cayenne, and a little bit of curry.
Shrimp to garnish the dish with.

Puree the fish in a food processor.
    Mix with spices, eggs, and cream, and puree longer.
    Transfer the mix into a buttered pan and cover with foil.
    Cook in a water bath at 350°F (175°C). It takes about 1 hour.
    Turn the pan over onto a serving plate and decorate with shrimp.

This dish is very rich. One 7 oz (200 g) serving of the mousse contains 500 calories and less than 3 grams of carbohydrates. If you serve it with a portion of my classic shrimp sauce (see page 160), you'll get a meal with 700 calories and a fat-burning quotient of 1.7. My shrimp sauce adds about 1 gram of carbohydrates per $\frac{2}{5}$ cup (100 ml) sauce. If you wish to lower the carbohydrate value and increase the fat-burning quotient, you can serve the pike and salmon mousse with melted butter instead of the sauce.

Fish and bacon

In Norway, it is common to eat pork and fish together. It is an excellent combination flavor-wise, as well as health-wise. You can sauté or boil the fish and serve it with bacon, butter, and horseradish, or you could sauté the fish together with the pork. Fish and bacon have about the same cooking time, but if you are using fresh pork, you should pre-sauté it.

The following is a nice recipe that I found online:

Sauté diced pork and onion in butter.
   Place a few fish fillets in a buttered ovenproof dish.
   Season with coarsely ground black pepper and some salt, if you want. Bacon usually provides enough salt.
   Pour the diced bacon and onions over the fish. Try adding chopped parsley and a few extra dabs of butter. If you want, grate some fresh horseradish on top.
   Cook at 350–400°F (175–200°C).

Serve with creamed spinach (see page 145), or some other delicious vegetable dish.
   This dish is very filling. 200 grams of bacon and fish with 200 grams creamed spinach provide about 900 calories and about 4 grams of carbohydrates. The fat-burning quotient is almost 2.

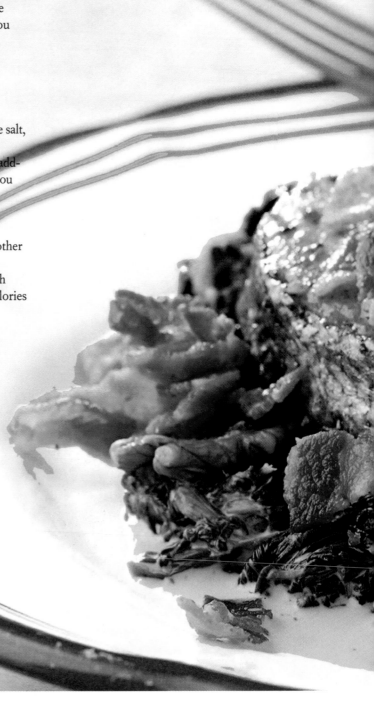

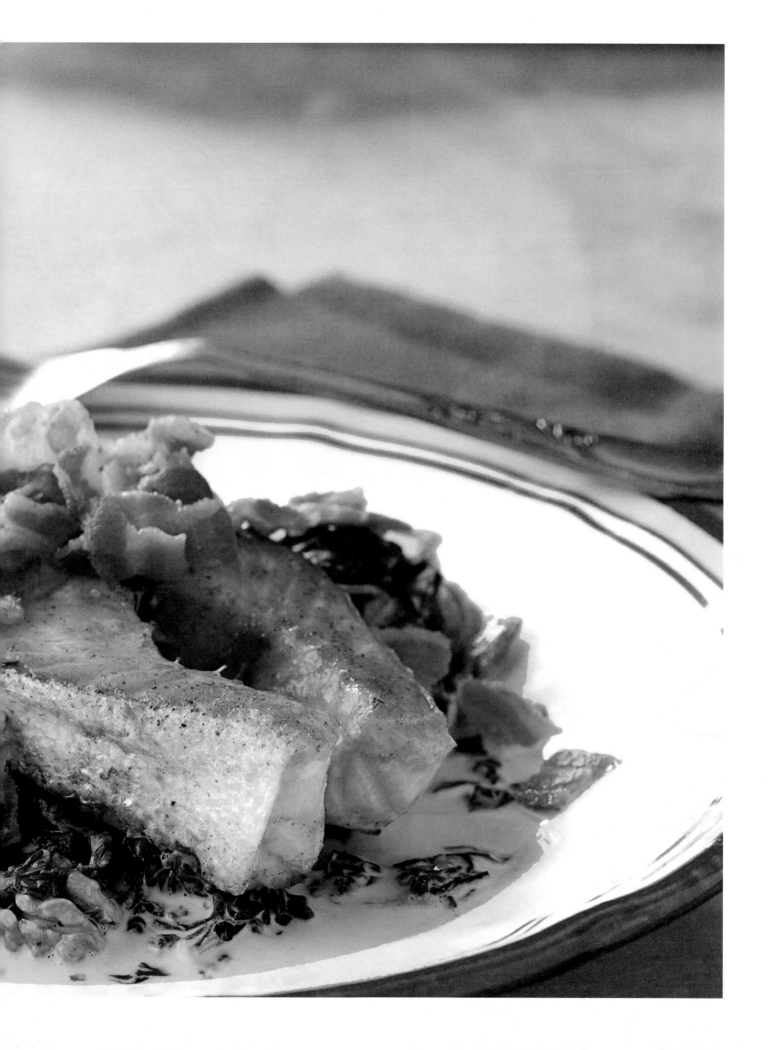

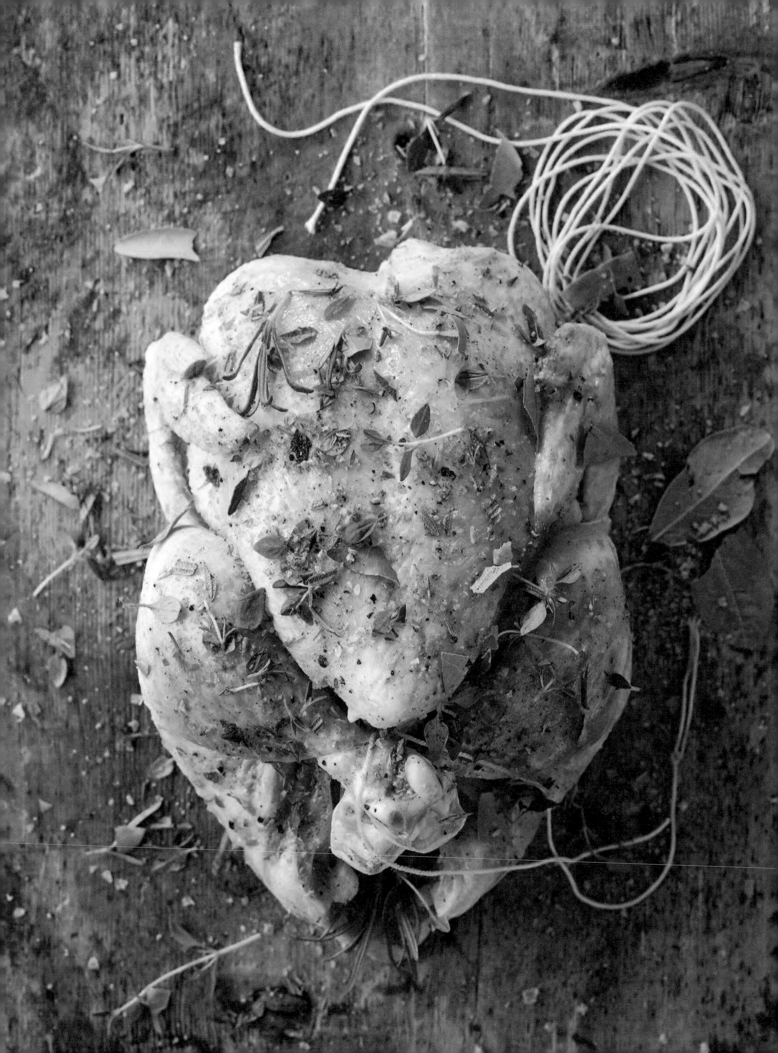

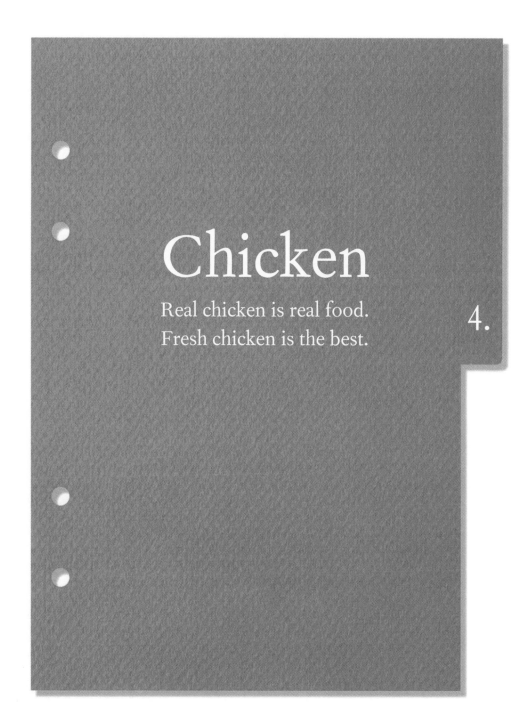

Chicken

Real chicken is real food.
Fresh chicken is the best.

4.

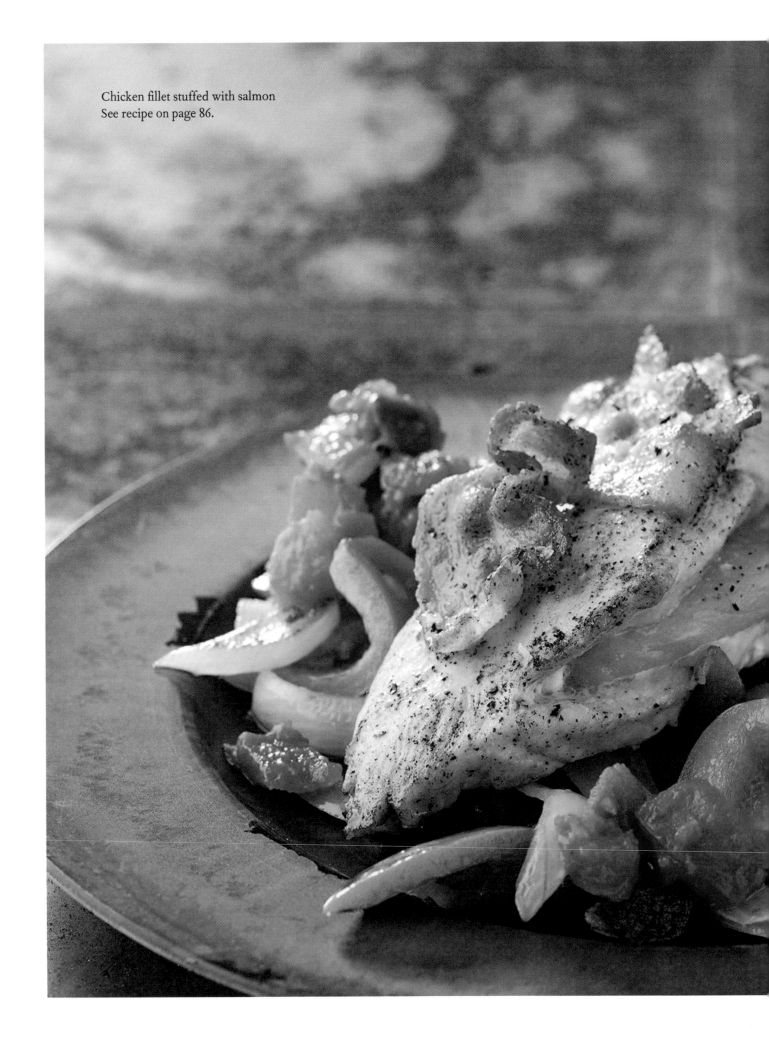

Chicken fillet stuffed with salmon
See recipe on page 86.

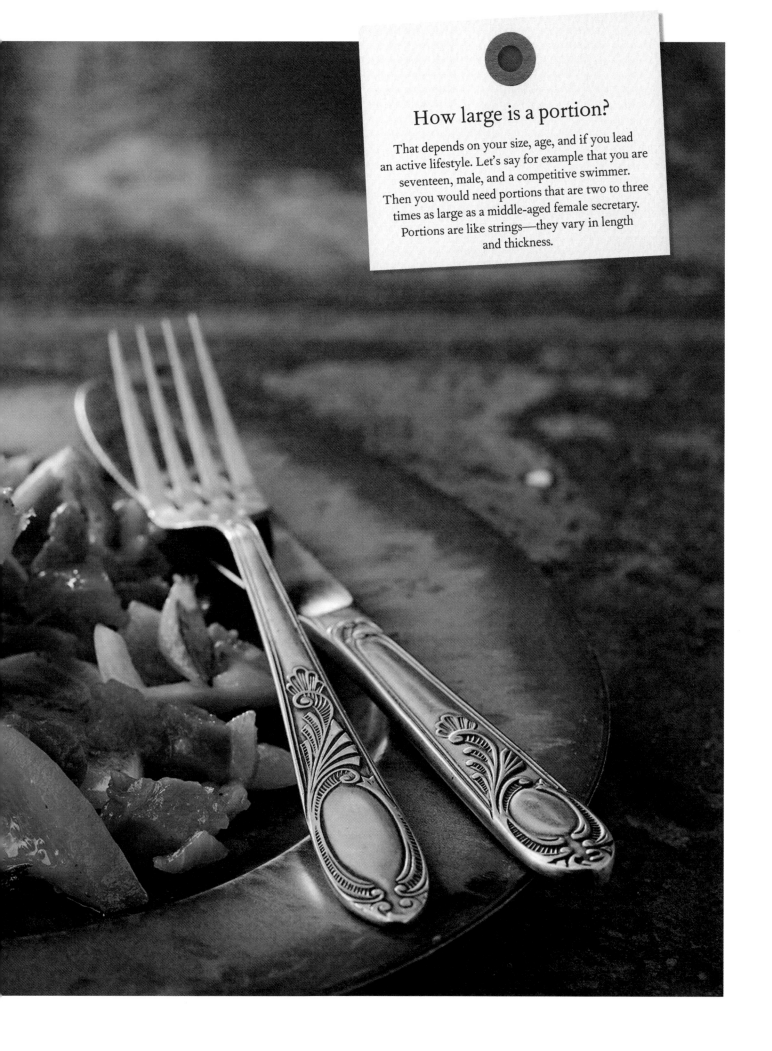

How large is a portion?

That depends on your size, age, and if you lead an active lifestyle. Let's say for example that you are seventeen, male, and a competitive swimmer. Then you would need portions that are two to three times as large as a middle-aged female secretary. Portions are like strings—they vary in length and thickness.

Chicken fillet stuffed with salmon

See photo on page 84.

1 chicken fillet per person, preferably with the skin
0.7 oz (20 g) bacon
One slice smoked salmon

Fill the chicken fillet with salmon, then fry it lightly in a skillet. Add bacon and butter on top of the fillet and transfer to the oven for about 20 minutes at 350°F (175°C).

For the side stir-fry:
1.8 oz (50 g) bacon
1 small yellow onion
1 shallot
2 cloves of garlic
About 10 oz (30 g) red, yellow, and green bell peppers
½ tablespoon ground coriander
1 tablespoon flavorful salsa, like yellow tomato and chili salsa

Fry the bacon in a wok, and take it out when it is cooked. Add the remaining ingredients for the side and fry them in the bacon fat. Add the bacon back in right before it is time to serve the dish.

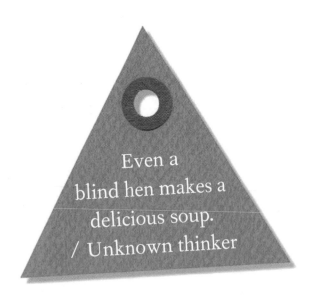

Even a blind hen makes a delicious soup. / Unknown thinker

Elisabet's chicken

A nice, large chicken is the most important component for this simple recipe. I recommend a corn-fed chicken. Corn is a form of grass, and while grass seeds aren't good human food, they are excellent as chicken feed. Let the birds eat the grass seeds, and then we can eat the birds; that's one of my mottos. Be meticulous when you choose your chicken. The frozen fillets injected with water that cost close to nothing are tasteless and unworthy food. No; you want an entire chicken, and fresh on top of that! A few years ago, you had to go to a market hall to get a good chicken. Now the yellow, delicious, corn-fed chickens are available at many grocery stores. Choose a nice big bird that weighs at least 3 pounds (about 1.5 kg).

A nice corn-fed chicken
Butter
Lemon
Salt and pepper
Vegetables of your choice
Heavy whipping cream and/or crème fraiche (for the sauce)

Cut up the chicken if you want, and rub the pieces with lemon, salt, and pepper. Cover with a few slices of butter. Roast the chicken whole for a fancier look. Elisabet roasts it at 350°F (175°C) for about an hour. When the chicken is close to being done, she adds heavy whipping cream and/or crème fraiche to the fatty chicken gravy. You can also add your vegetables at this point. Sometimes we use sugar snap peas and tomatoes, blanched nettles, or sautéed mushrooms. Continue to roast the chicken in the oven, then place it on the table.

Chicken meat without the skin is very lean, but this corn-fed chicken is fattier and delicious.

The carbohydrate value will vary depending on what sides you are serving with it. If you stick to only the chicken with the sauce, you'll get about 2–3 carbohydrates per serving. With the sugar snap peas, you'll increase the carbohydrate value to about 8–9 grams. Fat-burning quotient: 1.5.

Appropriate sides: Mashed cauliflower is an excellent choice for this dish (see recipe on page 146).

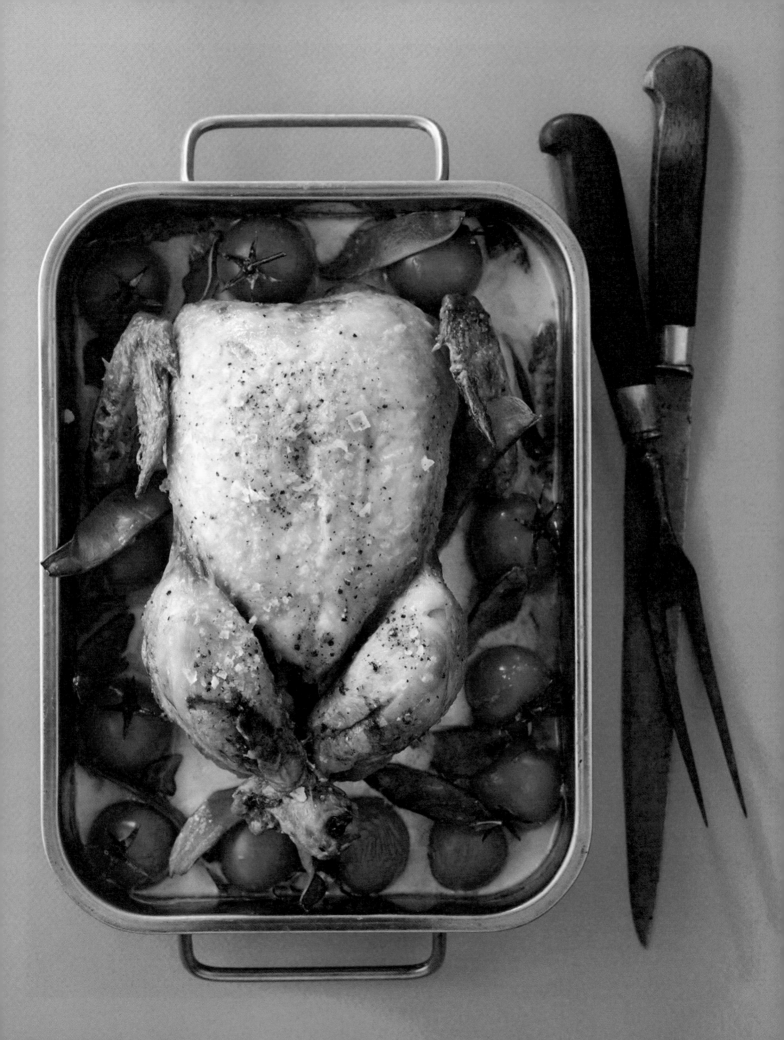

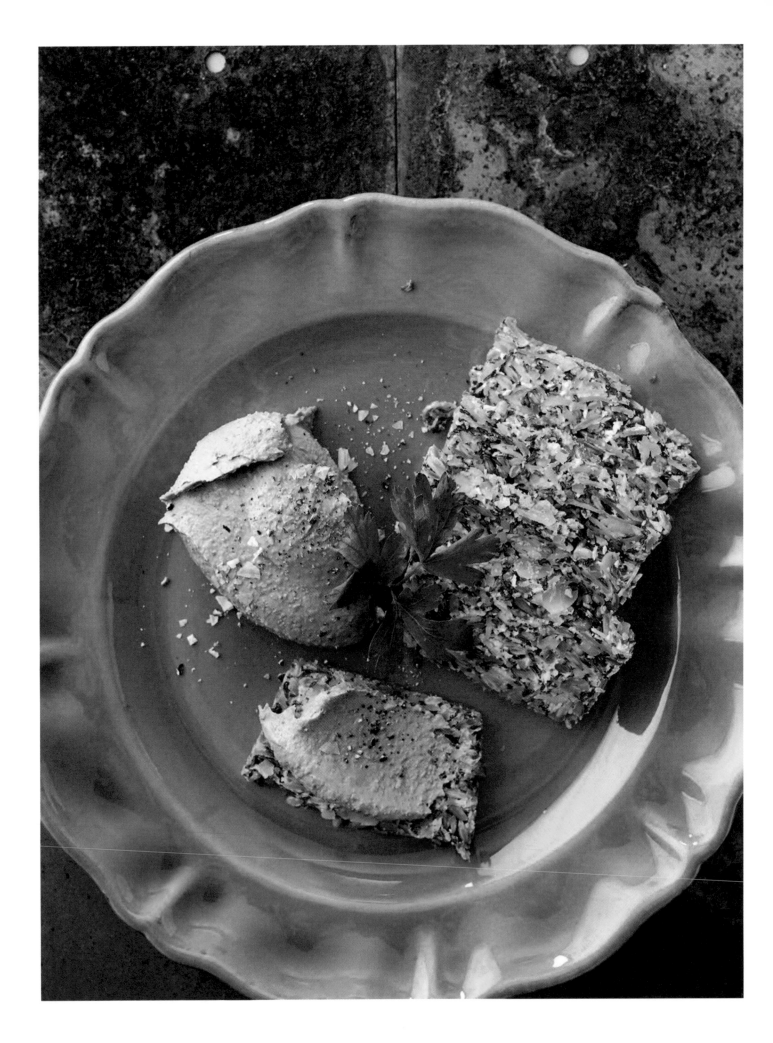

"Grass seeds, such as barley, wheat, rye, and corn, are bird food. Let the birds fatten up on bird food, then we can eat the birds. The same reasoning can be applied to cows."
/SSS

Maggan's chicken liver mousse

Liver is probably one of the healthiest foods we can consume. No other food contains as many vitamins and minerals as liver. Those who think that fruits and vegetables contain a lot of nutrients should compare an apple to liver. Try feeding the values into a computer-based nutritional program. An apple contains sugar, water, and a little bit of vitamin C. Compare that to beef liver. The nutrition value goes through the roof!

People who don't like the taste of sautéed liver can consume liver pâté instead. The better option is always to make your own pâté or mousse from scratch. The following is a quick and simple recipe.

8.8 oz (400 g) chicken liver
3.5–7 oz (100–200 g) butter
⅘ cup (200 ml) heavy whipping cream
Salt and spices

Sauté the chicken liver in plenty of butter until it is thoroughly cooked. (The liver will cook faster if you cut it into smaller pieces).

Season with salt and pepper and add other spices according to your own preference (I use herb seasoning and garlic).

Mix the sautéed liver with the heavy whipping cream in a food processor; you can also add some extra butter and spices.

Taste and season more if needed until you are satisfied with the flavor. Pour the batter into a buttered pan that you can cover with a lid. The batter will be pretty runny, but don't worry, the pâté will solidify in the fridge.

The original recipe makes a pâté with the usual consistency of liver pâté, but without the additives. Perfect at any occasions where you would normally serve pâté.

If we make four servings out of this pâté, each portion contains 500–600 calories, depending on the amount of butter used. Each portion has about 2.4 grams of carbohydrates and a fat burning quotient that is a little bit higher than 2. Chicken liver contains the least carbohydrates of all types of liver, so it is a wise choice for anyone who is looking to lose weight.

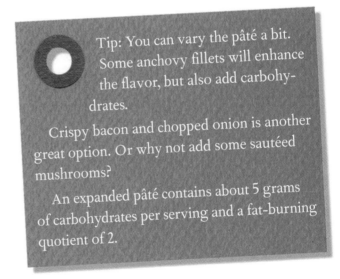

Tip: You can vary the pâté a bit. Some anchovy fillets will enhance the flavor, but also add carbohydrates.

Crispy bacon and chopped onion is another great option. Or why not add some sautéed mushrooms?

An expanded pâté contains about 5 grams of carbohydrates per serving and a fat-burning quotient of 2.

Boiled chicken

A fine chicken should boil in its own broth, not broth made from a cube (and definitely not in water!). If you happen to have chicken broth in the freezer, use it. If not, make one from the leftover chicken pieces; follow the recipe for the chicken soup on page 31. This will of course make the meal a lot more time-consuming than if you already have homemade broth in the freezer.

Roughly chop the chicken breast lengthwise and cross-wise, or however you want to cut it up, and simmer the pieces together with the chicken thighs in the broth. Remove the pot from the heat and pour some of the cooking liquid into a small saucepan. The broth should cook until about half of it evaporates, so you'll need at least 17 oz (½ liter) of broth for two people. This sauce is popular!

While the broth is simmering, get the sides ready. Personally, I love haricot verts, spinach, or asparagus (see recipe on page 145). I usually cook them quickly in salted water with butter, then I turn off the heat and leave them in the hot liquid.

Once the base for the sauce is cooked, I add ⅖ cup (100 ml) heavy whipping cream, or ⅘ cup (200 ml) if I have a lot of broth. I season the sauce with whatever I feel like that day, usually *sambal oelek* (sometimes curry), and perhaps a few drops of lemon juice and some pepper. Salt is usually not needed. At the end, I thicken the sauce with some egg yolks that I've mixed with cream. Count on about 2 yolks per person.

Heat the chicken pieces and serve with the sauce and vegetables.

Nutritional value: One portion of boiled chicken contains nearly zero grams of carbohydrates, but the meat is packed with proteins and contains hardly any fat. The sauce contains about 1 gram per ⅖ cup (100 ml). The vegetables pass the carbohydrate test with about 1–3 grams of carbs per 3.5 oz (1 hg), and the spinach contains the least amount. That's fewer than 4 grams of carbohydrates in total for a hearty meal with chicken, sauce, and spinach. If you choose haricot verts, you'll add about 2 more grams per serving. The fat-burning quotient is just below 1, depending on the high protein content.

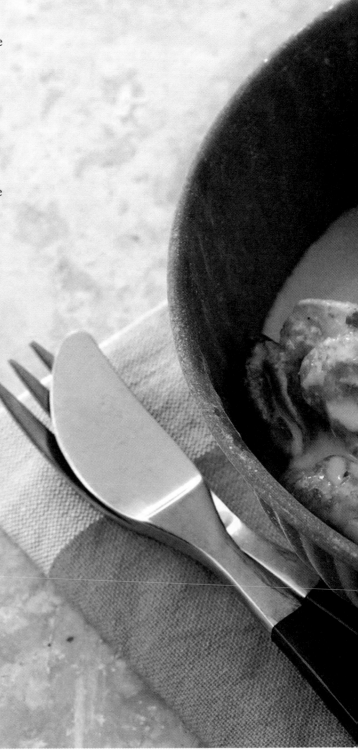

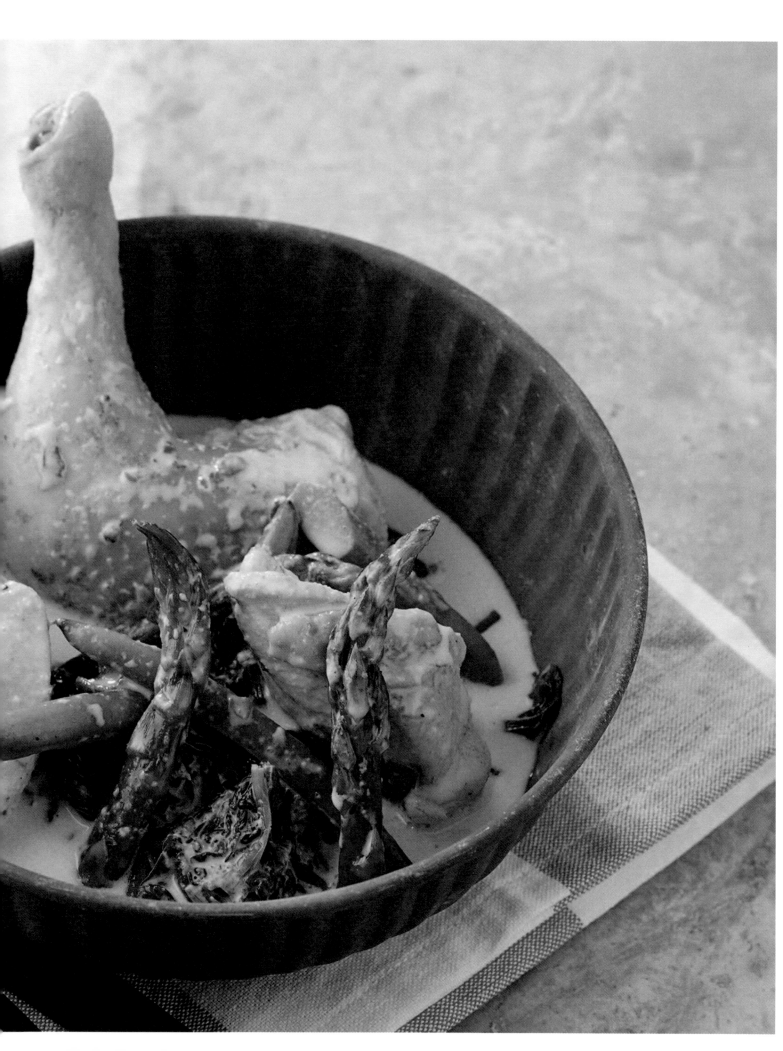

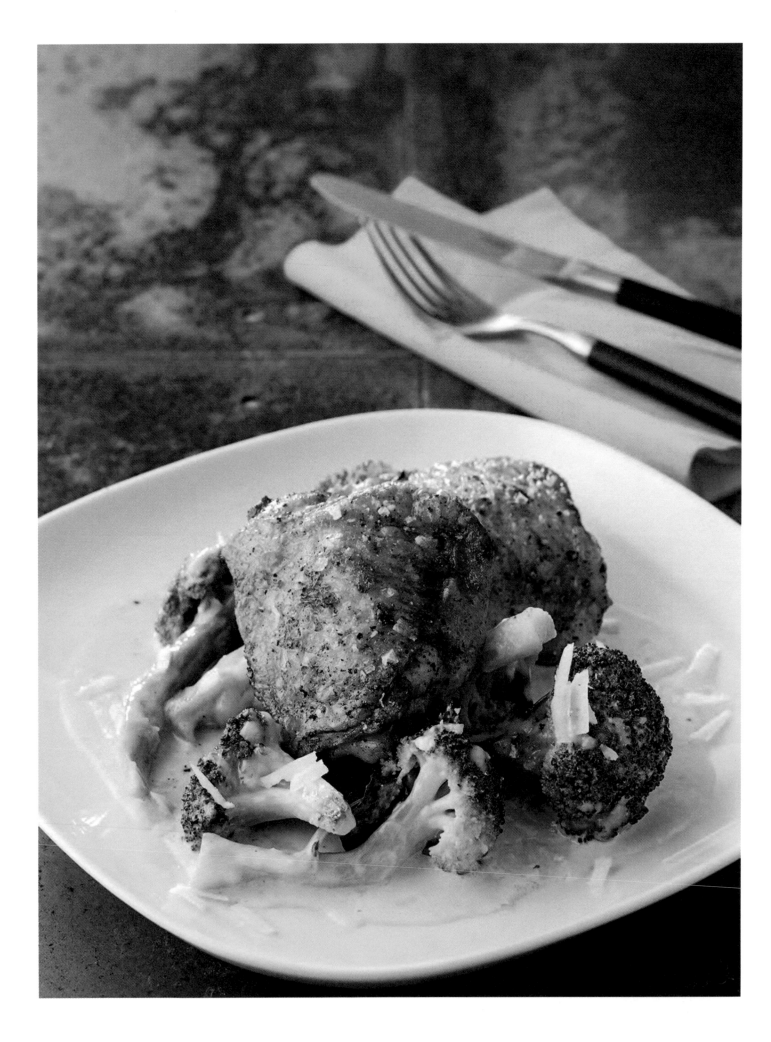

Cognac chicken with Parmesan broccoli

I found this recipe online. Whoever signed the recipe as "Asami," somehow made a meal that is completely up my alley. She wrote:

"Tried something new yesterday with ingredients that I happened to have at home. It turned out absolutely delicious, and I just have to share it with you!"

For the chicken:
Sauté chicken thighs (or whatever parts you prefer) in a skillet on fairly high heat so that the pieces turn out really crispy. Season with plenty of black pepper and salt. Add about ⅖ cup (100 ml) or more of cognac, cover with a lid, and simmer until the chicken is cooked.

For the broccoli:
In a skillet, sauté broccoli florets in butter. When the broccoli has softened a little, add some cream and continue cooking the broccoli florets until they are done. Press a garlic clove, or two, into the cream. Grate a generous amount of Parmesan cheese and sprinkle it over the broccoli at the end. Any other seasoning is barely needed. Once the cheese has melted, the dish is ready.

A hefty portion with two parts meat and one part broccoli contains about 5 grams of carbohydrates (mostly from the broccoli). The fat-burning quotient is 0.75. If you are using Västerbotten cheese instead of Parmesan, the fat-burning quotient is 0.8.

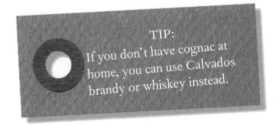
TIP:
If you don't have cognac at home, you can use Calvados, brandy or whiskey instead.

Chicken fillet gratin with salsa

See photo on page 94.

In my house, we always cook delicious meals by throwing together whatever we may have at home that day. Today, my wife cooked, and dinner was a huge success. Naturally, I have to share the recipe in this book.

4 fine chicken breast fillets, each 7 oz (200 g)
Butter, oil, salt, and pepper

For the sauce:
⅖ cup (100 ml) yogurt/cream (alternatively, ⅖ cup (100 ml) crème fraiche)
⅖ cup (100 g) grated Parmesan
3–4 sundried tomatoes in oil, chopped
2 crushed garlic cloves

This is a very simple and easy-to-make dish. The idea is to brown the chicken fillets, then finish cooking them in the oven with the sauce, and serve with sides of your choice.

Preheat the oven to 400°F (200°C), and begin making the sauce, if you haven't made it in advance. I usually keep a jar of it in the fridge. Flatten the chicken fillets and sauté them in a blend of butter and oil. Season with salt and pepper. Brown the fillets thoroughly and keep them on the hot stove for a little bit afterwards. They should be cooked almost all the way through. While the chicken sits on the stove, mix the sauce to cover the chicken with.

Transfer the chicken fillets to an ovenproof dish and cover them with the sauce. Check on the dish after 15 minutes and remove it from the oven once it has a nice color. It should take 20 minutes at the most.

My wife cooked this dish in about 30 minutes. However, she already had the sauce ready in the fridge. We ate one chicken fillet each, and about the equal amount of sides, and it more than satisfied our appetite.

In other words, the food would have been enough for four people. My portion contained about 1,000 calories and about 10 grams of carbohydrates. The fat-burning quotient was about 1.3. The nutritional value was good too, with two and a half times the daily recommended value of saturated fat, and three-quarters of your day's worth of cholesterol. This meal is a great building block for the immune system.

Recommended side: Salsa (see recipe on page 147).

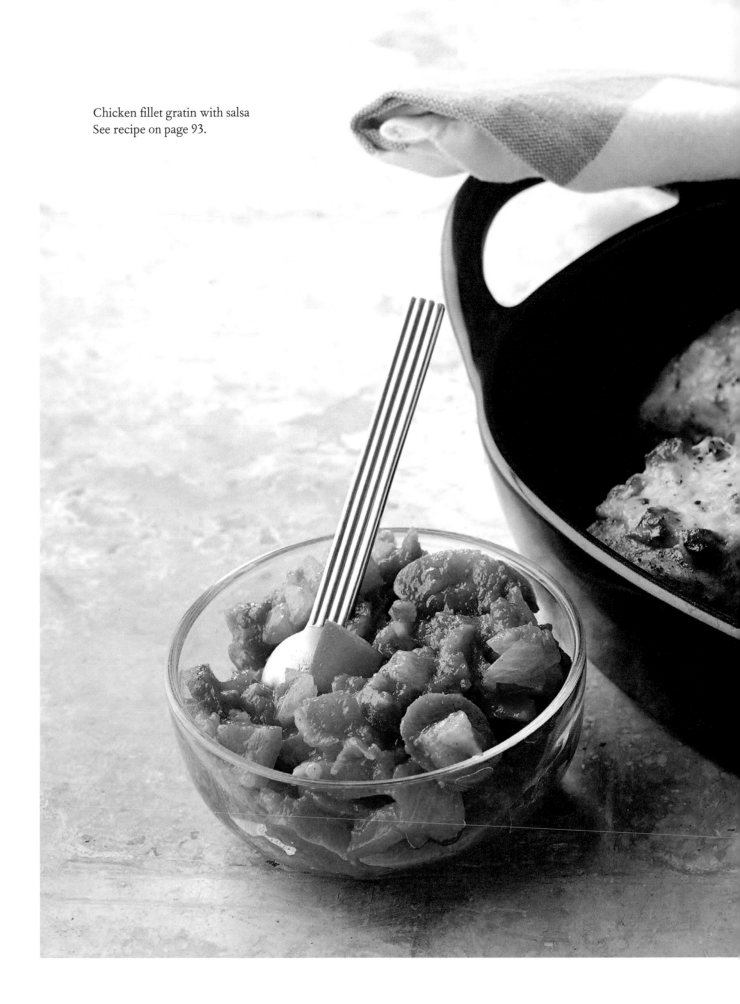

Chicken fillet gratin with salsa
See recipe on page 93.

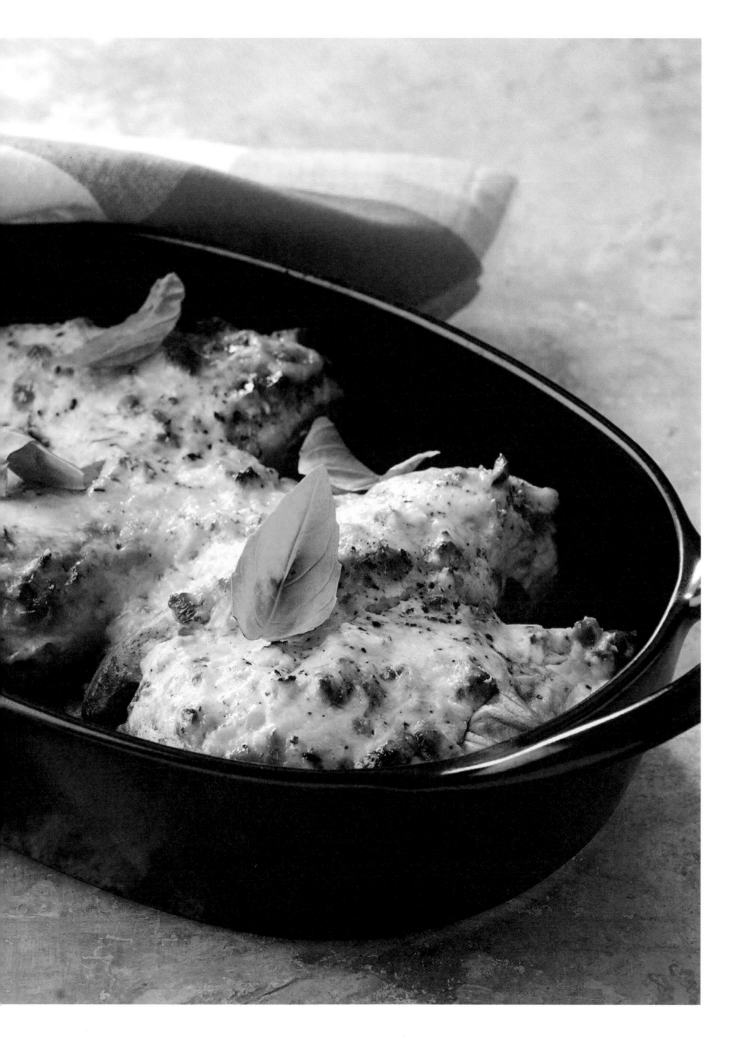

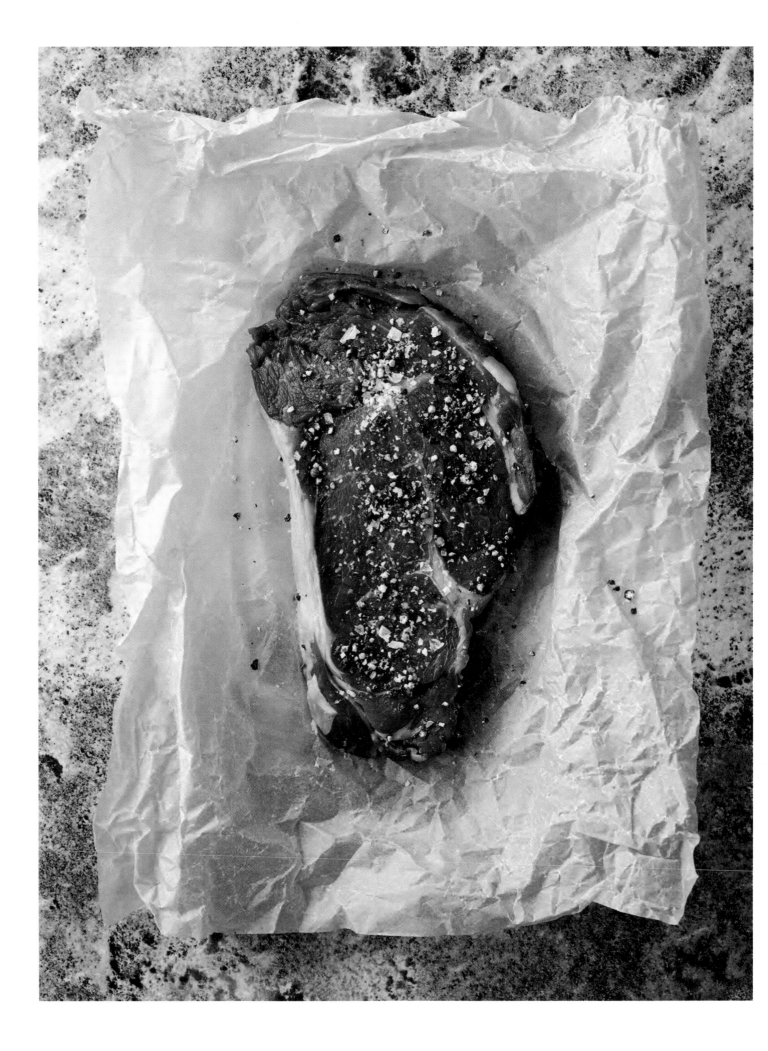

Meat

We are designed to
eat meat from animals that
have lived a natural life.

5.

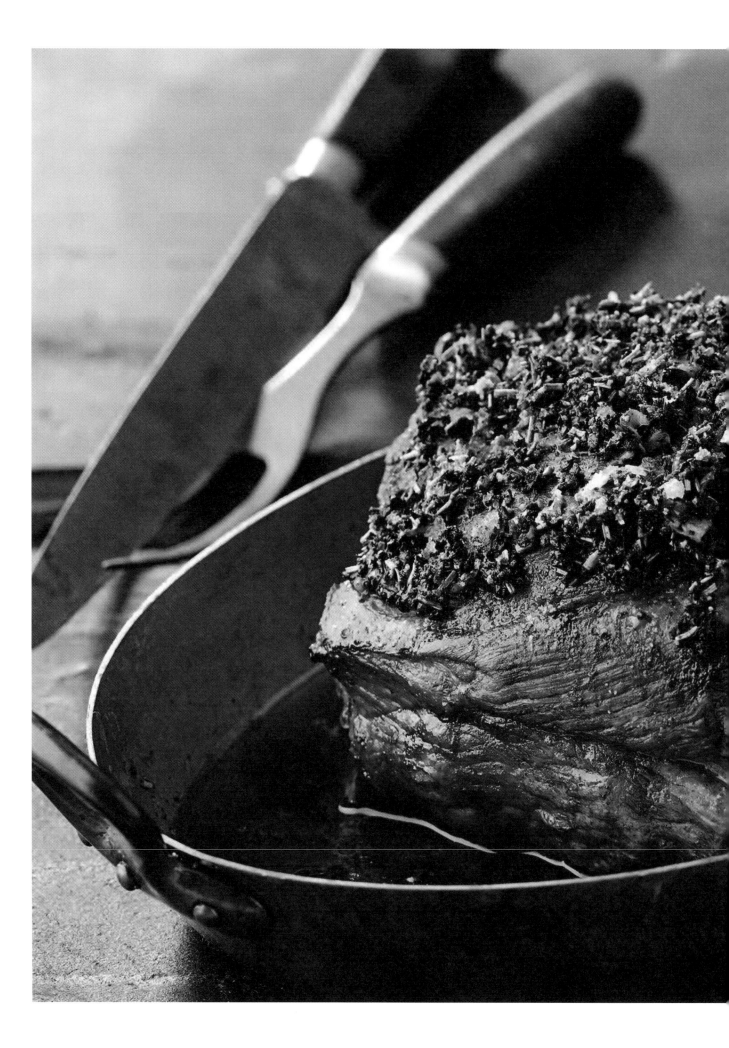

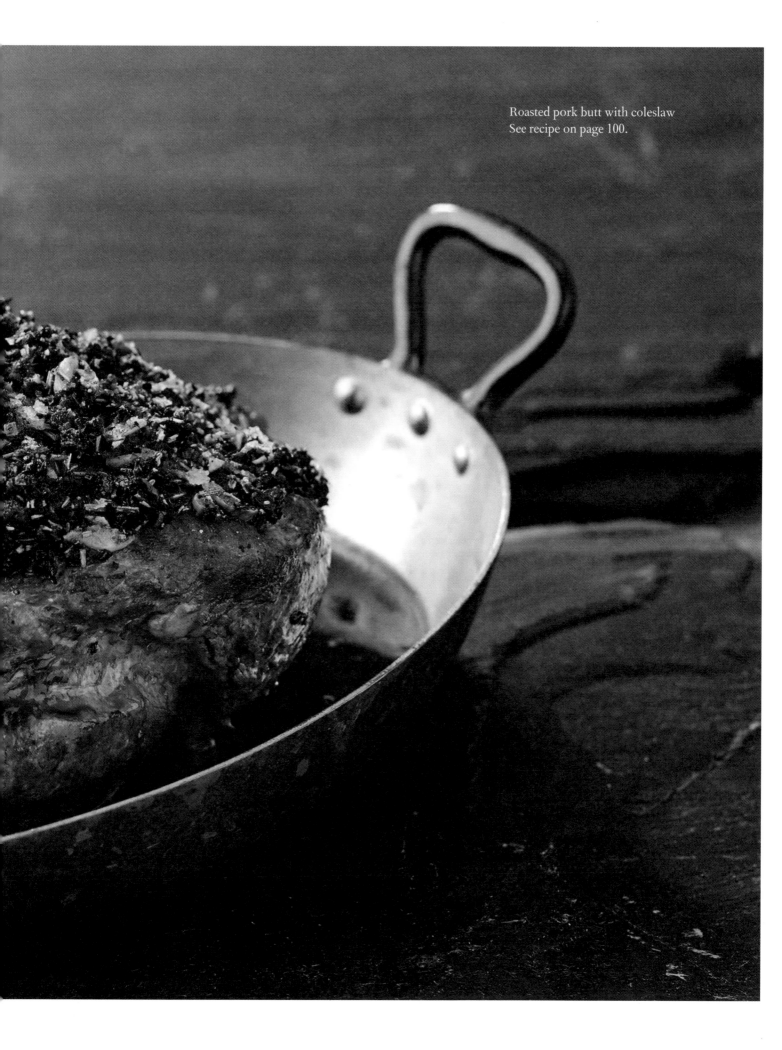

Roasted pork butt with coleslaw
See recipe on page 100.

"Mostly eat what has moved. And let the food hang for a while. Sixty days is about enough. If the food is still screaming after that, it hasn't been hanging long enough."

/SSS

Roasted pork butt with coleslaw

See photo on page 98.

Pork butt in pieces, about 2.2 lbs (1 kg)

Butter and olive oil

⅕ cup (50 g) tapenade

A few sprigs of rosemary, or 1 tablespoon dried rosemary

2–3 cloves of garlic

Salt and black pepper

Brown the pork butt in butter and olive oil.
    Season with salt and black pepper.
    Mix tapenade, crushed garlic cloves, and finely chopped rosemary.
    Spread the mix over the browned pork butt and transfer the meat to the oven at 300°F (150°C). I usually remove the meat from the oven and pack it in aluminum foil once it reaches an inner temperature of 167°F (75°C). The meat will reach 175°F (80°C) after 15 minutes.

Serve with coleslaw (see recipe on page 147). One serving of pork butt with a dollop of coleslaw contains about 700 calories and about 4–5 grams of carbohydrates. The fat-burning quotient is about 1.3. If you want to improve the fat-burning quotient, add more coleslaw to the portion; just be aware that this will also add some carbohydrates to the meal.

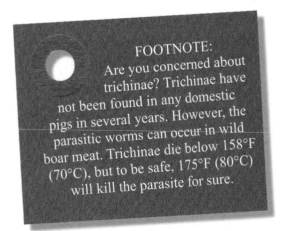

FOOTNOTE:
Are you concerned about trichinae? Trichinae have not been found in any domestic pigs in several years. However, the parasitic worms can occur in wild boar meat. Trichinae die below 158°F (70°C), but to be safe, 175°F (80°C) will kill the parasite for sure.

Stuffed pork tenderloin

It is always a good idea to stuff meat with something flavorful. This is what my sister-in-law, Kristina, does with her pork tenderloin.

1 pork tenderloin, about 1.1–2.2 lbs (½–1 kg)

Butter for sautéing

For the stuffing:

Sundried tomatoes, sparse amount

Mozzarella

Pesto, generous amount

Basil

Black pepper (no salt needed)

Bacon (1 package) to wrap around the stuffed fillet

Cut up the fillet so that you can spread out a flat piece—kind of like when you make a jelly roll, but backwards. If this is too difficult, just make an incision in the meat.
    Mix sundried tomatoes with sliced mozzarella, pesto, basil, and black pepper, and spread the blend over the meat. Be generous.
    Roll the meat tightly and wrap in bacon. Secure with a cotton string and season with more black pepper.
    Brown the roll in butter in a skillet.
    Roast the meat in the oven at 350–400°F (175–200°C) until it is cooked. It takes about 45 minutes.

Recommended sides: Green salad (see recipe on page 39).

One serving of stuffed fillet that weighs about 7 oz (200 g) contains fewer than 600 calories and 4–5 grams of carbohydrates. The fat-burning quotient is about 0.8. Choose vegetables according to your own preference and needs. If you eat this meal with coleslaw, the fat-burning quotient goes up to 1.1.

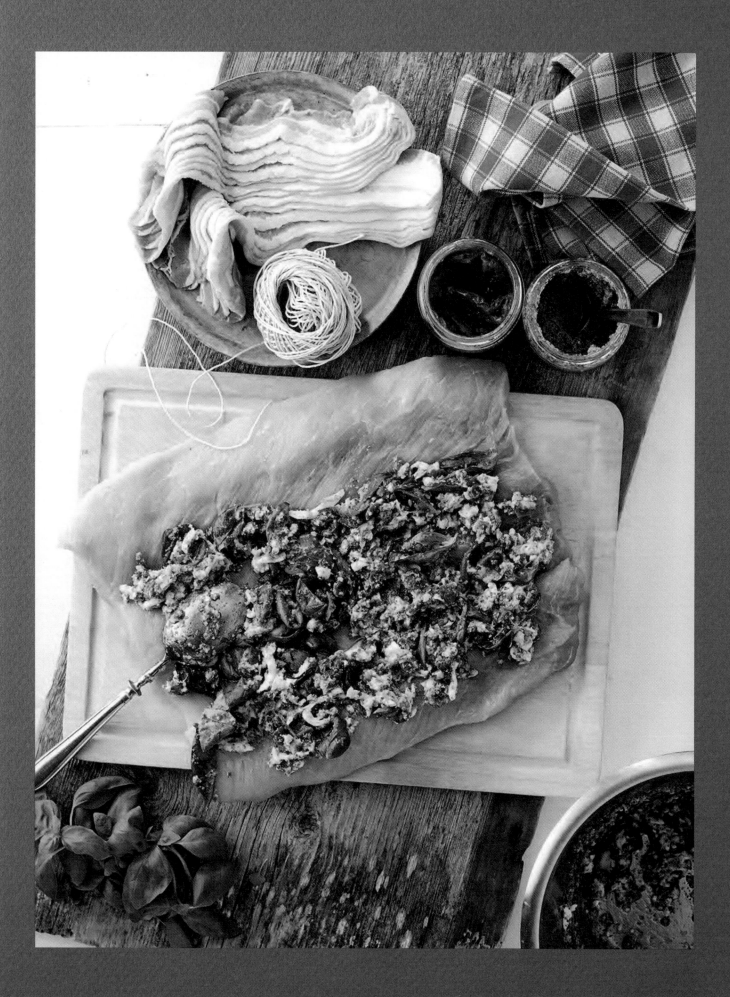

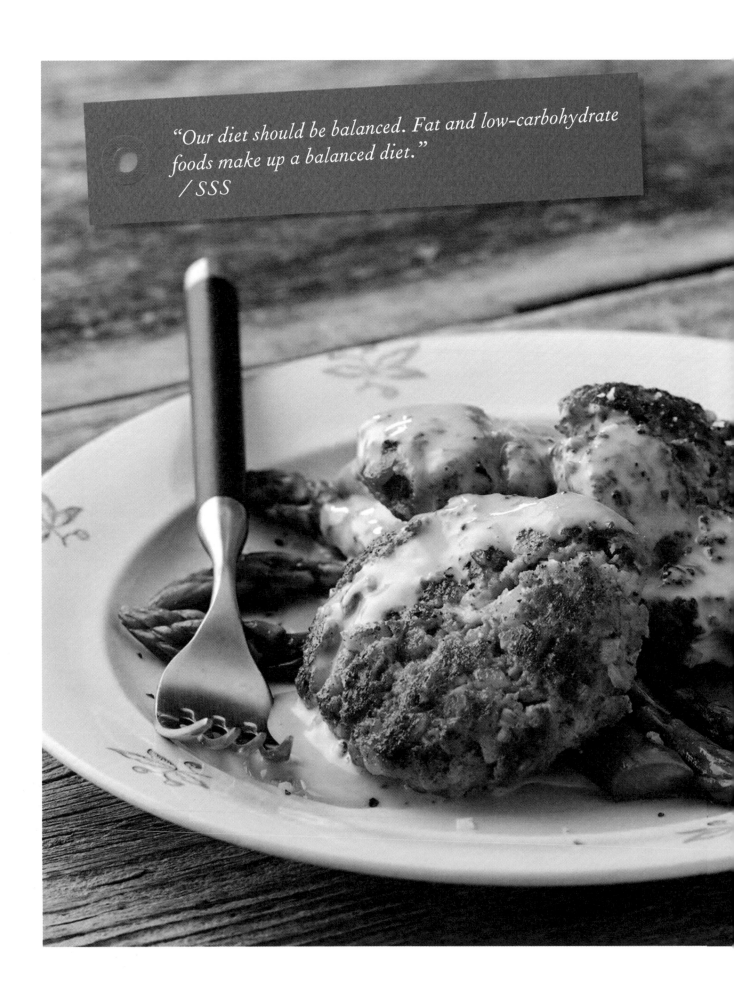

"*Our diet should be balanced. Fat and low-carbohydrate foods make up a balanced diet.*"
/ SSS

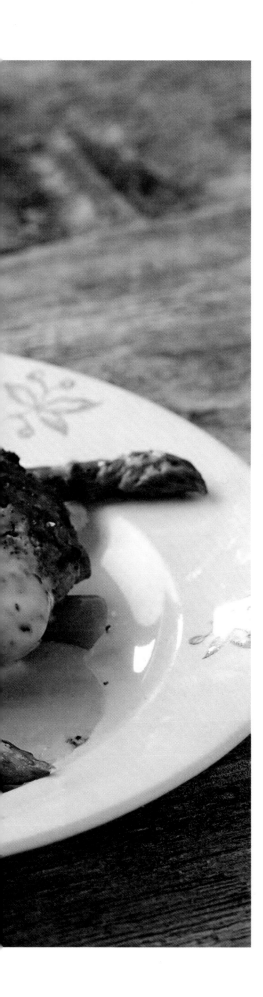

Ground lamb with bacon

Ground meat dishes should always be cooked in massive amounts. Never make less than two pounds. If you are going to bother with making a mess, you may as well get a lot out of that mess. Personally, I love ground lamb.

2.2 lbs (1 kg) ground lamb
1–2 packages of finely chopped and crispy bacon
Asparagus
1 yellow onion, finely chopped
²⁄₅ cup (100 ml) heavy whipping cream
2 eggs
½ tablespoon Dijon mustard (optional)
1 package crumbled feta cheese, or 7 oz (200 g) grated cheese
Butter and olive oil for sautéing
Heavy whipping cream and Japanese soy sauce for the sauce

Cook the bacon until crispy, and cook a vegetable of your choice. I always love asparagus. (Otherwise, I love to eat this ground lamb dish with coleslaw; find the recipe on page 147.) Once the bacon has cooled, mix all the ingredients together, season, and sauté for a little while. Keep in mind that the bacon and feta cheese both contain quite a bit of salt!

If you are satisfied with the flavor, shape the mix into flat balls, sauté them and place on warm plates. Cook the heavy whipping cream in a skillet. A teaspoon of Japanese soy sauce will add flavor to the sauce. Increase the heat and bring to a boil. It only takes about a minute.

This dish is great for anyone who is trying to lose weight. 7 oz (200 g) of the ground lamb, with ⅕ cup (50 ml) of cream sauce, only contain about 600 calories and 3 grams of carbohydrates. The fat-burning quotient is about 1.5. If you serve it with 2.5 oz (70 g) of asparagus and a tablespoon of butter, you'll raise the meal to 700 calories and barely 5 grams of carbohydrates. What a pleasurable meal for whoever wants to lose weight!

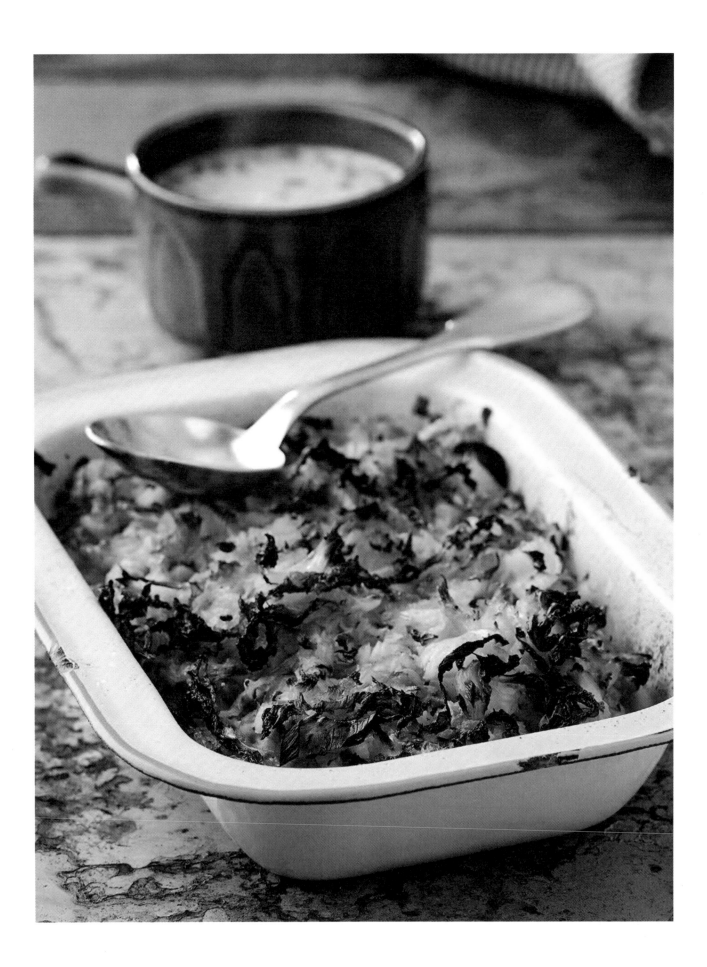

Cabbage pudding

Cabbage is delicious and healthy, and it contains a fairly small number of carbohydrates. See my carbohydrate table on page 13. I enjoy cabbage soup, mutton in cabbage, and cabbage pudding. Not to mention cabbage salads!

I got this recipe from an old friend of mine, Karen Pilgaard.

28 oz (800 g) white cabbage, or savoy cabbage
1 small leek (optional)
2–3 tablespoons butter
⅖ cup (100 ml) water
Salt and white pepper

For the ground meat:
17.5 oz (500 g) mix of ground beef and pork
2 yellow onions, chopped
2 eggs
⅖ cup (100 ml) heavy whipping cream
1 teaspoon salt
Coarsely ground black pepper (according to your own preference)

For the cream sauce:
1⅓ cups (300 ml) heavy whipping cream
1 broth cube
Salt, white pepper
A little bit of soy sauce if you want
2–3 tablespoons fresh or frozen lingon berries

Shred or chop the cabbage and the leek. Sauté them in butter and season with salt and pepper. Dilute with water and simmer for 10–15 minutes. Allow to cool off for a little bit.

Bring the ingredients for the sauce to a boil and serve with the pudding.

Lingon berries are great as a side to this dish.
Count on about 4 servings for this cabbage pudding. Each portion contains about 800 calories and about 13–14 carbohydrates. The fat burning quotient is 1.7. If you want fewer carbohydrates, just use less cabbage and add more meat to the pudding. You can also skip the leek. Then you'll get about 10 grams of carbohydrates per serving. You only need to lower the carbohydrates further if you are following a strict diet to lose weight.

Bolognese with zucchini pasta

See photo on page 106.
14–21 oz (400–600 g) ground meat (pork and beef mixed together, or just pork)
1 large onion
2–3 cloves of garlic
1 finely chopped chili (optional)
Butter or olive oil for sautéing
1 tablespoon tomato purée
½ package crushed tomatoes
Salt and pepper
Fond or Japanese soy sauce to add flavor
1 teaspoon oregano
⅘–1⅓ cups (200–300 ml) heavy whipping cream
Flavorful cheese of your choice, grated

Sauté the ground meat in butter and olive oil.

Push the meat to the side of the skillet, lower the heat, and add the chopped onion.

Once the onion has gotten some color, add the rest of the ingredients, stir, and cook the sauce.

Taste and adjust seasonings if needed.

Serve with zucchini pasta (see recipe on page 150). Sprinkle with grated cheese. A few leafy greens and a tomato wedge will add some nice color to the plate.

The meat sauce contains about 8 grams of carbohydrates and has a fat-burning quotient of about 1.5. Most of the carbohydrates come from the tomatoes, secondly from the onion, and at last from the heavy whipping cream.

The zucchini pasta adds about 3 grams of carbohydrates per 3.5 oz (1 hg) and increases the fat-burning quotient a few tenths. This is a great meal for anyone who isn't extremely carbohydrate sensitive.

Bolognese with zucchini pasta
See recipe on page 105.

"I often cook with wine, sometimes I even add it to the food."

/ W.C. Fields, Comedian

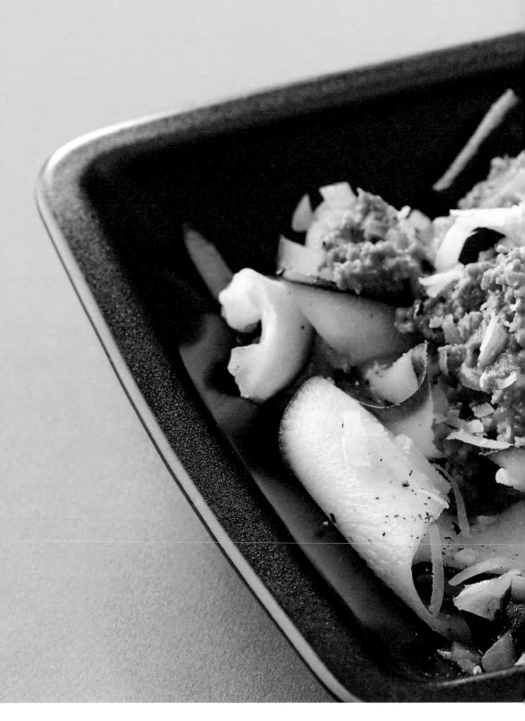

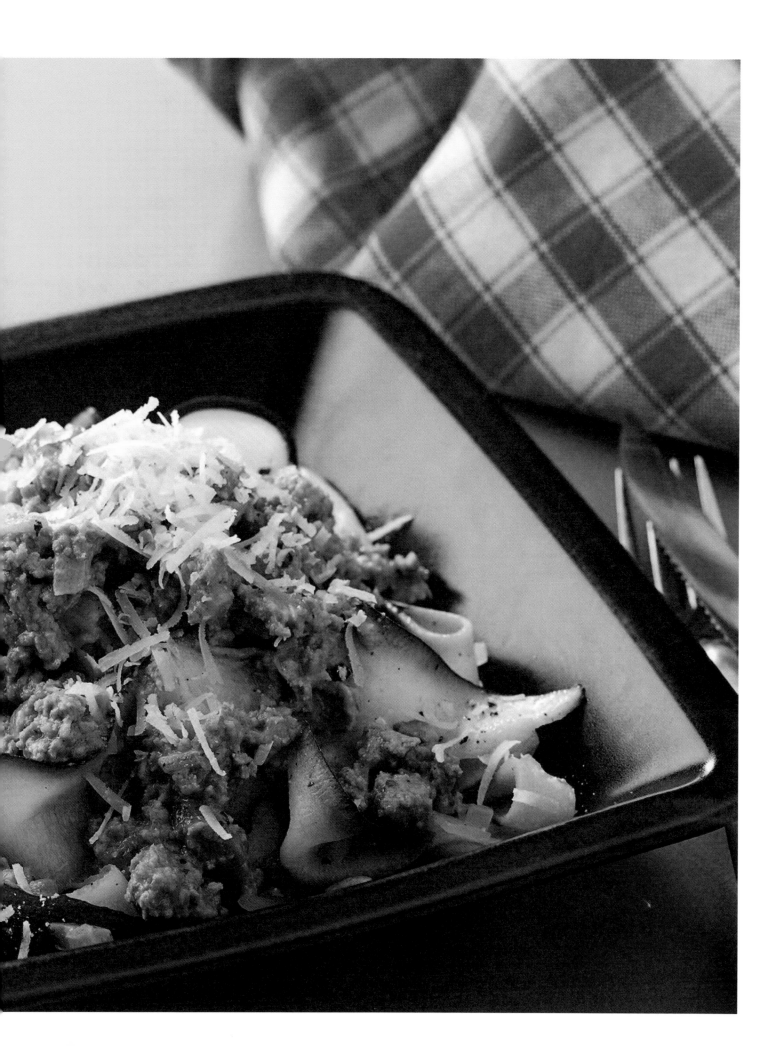

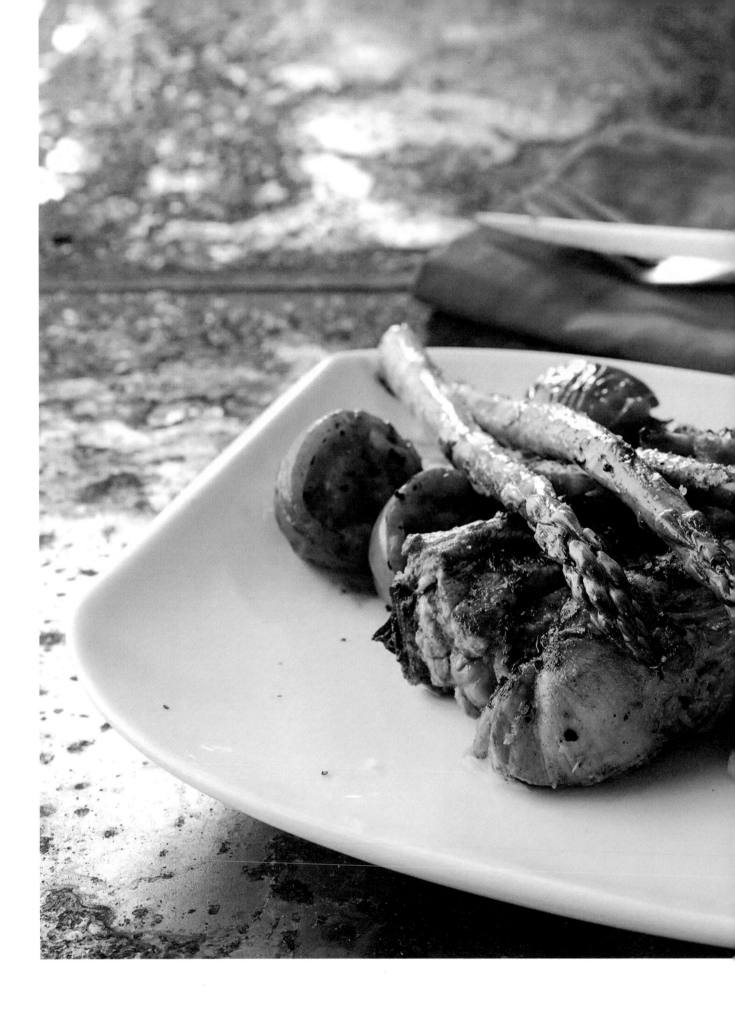

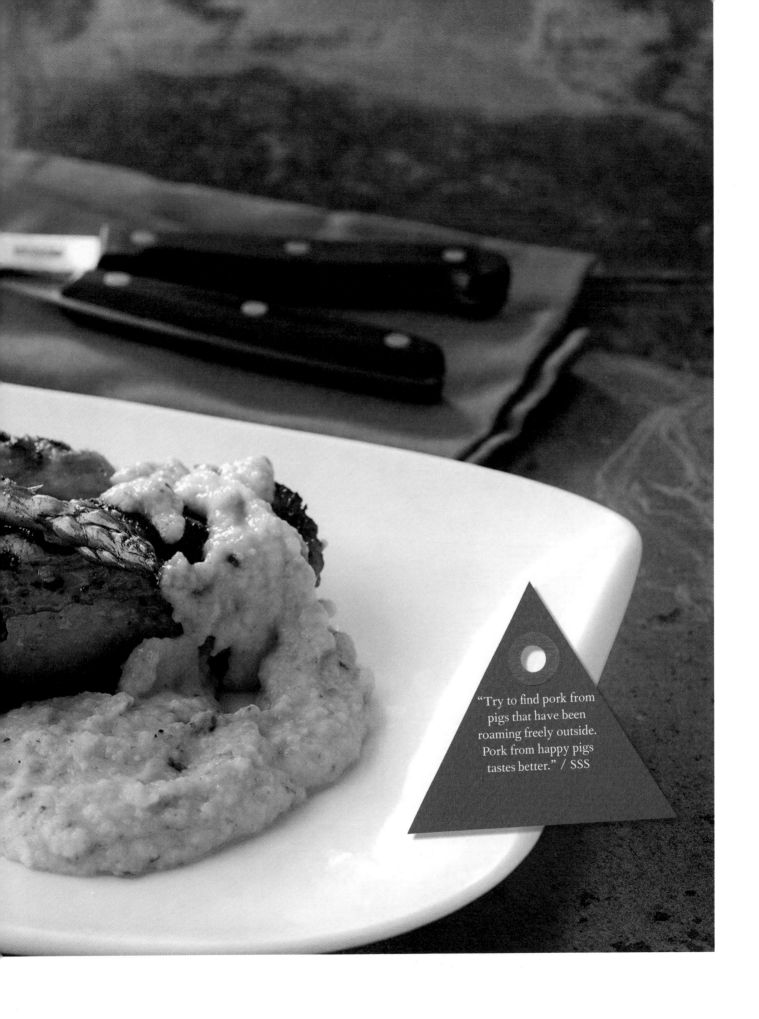

"Try to find pork from pigs that have been roaming freely outside. Pork from happy pigs tastes better." / SSS

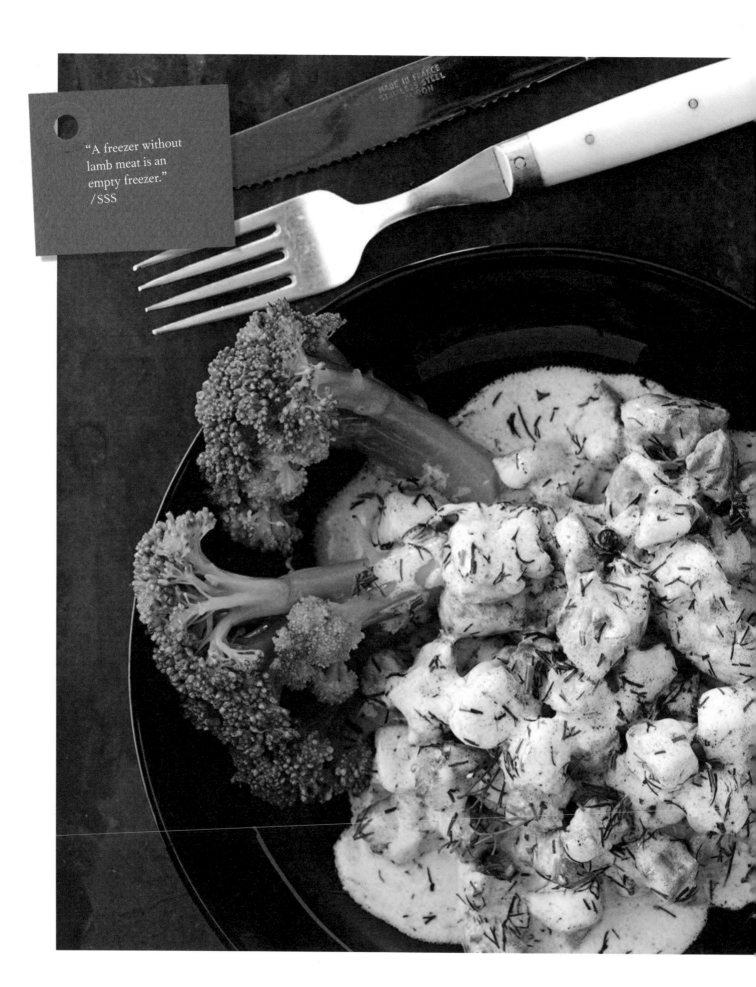

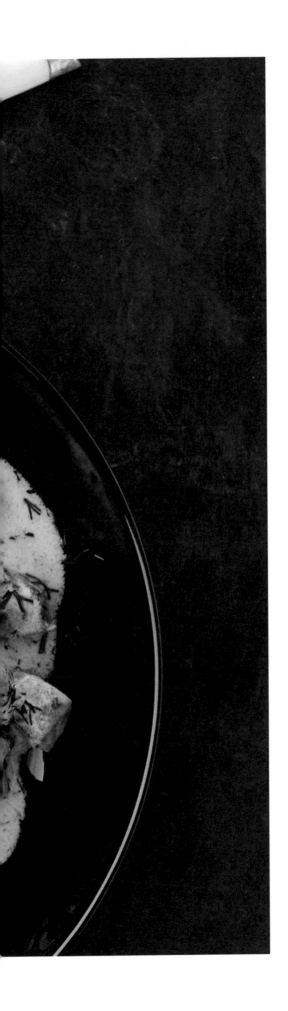

Pork loin cutlet with carrot béarnaise

See photo on page 109.

To switch out the traditional ribs, cook pork loin cutlets every once in a while. Not all grocery stores will offer that type of cut, but if you have a manual meat counter close by, you can quickly get pork loin cutlet row cut up, and folded out into a cutlet. Perfect on the grill and for the oven!

At least 14 oz (4 hg) pork loin cutlet per person
French mustard
Finely grated ginger
Salt and pepper
Butter

Generously rub the cutlet row with the remaining ingredients.
    Roast at 400°F (200°C) for about 1 hour.

Serve with carrot béarnaise (see recipe on page 159) and a nice vegetable.

This is a fairly lean and low-carbohydrate meal. Count on about 2 grams of carbohydrates per serving when it comes to the meat. Fat-burning quotient is about 1. You'll get a lot of healthy saturated fat, plenty of B-vitamins, and a nice composition of minerals. One serving of the carrot béarnaise adds about 4 grams of carbohydrates, and a little bit of butter-cooked broccoli will add some additional carbohydrates. Still, the meal contains below 10 grams of carbohydrates per serving and is a good option for anyone who is following a strict diet to lose weight.

Lamb in dill

A piece of boneless lamb meat (preferably brisket),
    count on about 4.2 oz (120 g) per person
Salt, pepper, allspice, and dill
Crème fraiche

Cut the meat into pieces, about 0.5–1 square inch each, and rub with pepper and salt. Brown on high heat for a few minutes. Boil down the skillet in between each round, and transfer the meat with added water if necessary. Add a few whole allspice berries. Simmer for about 1–1½ hours. Skim off the fat. Strain about ⅔ of the broth through a sieve. Add half of the dill for the last 30 minutes. Add the crème fraiche—about ⅖ cup (100 g) per person—and the remaining dill (it should be fresh). Simmer for about half an hour.

Recommended sides: Coleslaw (see recipe on page 147), or some sort of butter-cooked vegetable that grows above ground. The amount of carbohydrates will vary with whatever sides you chose to serve with this dish.

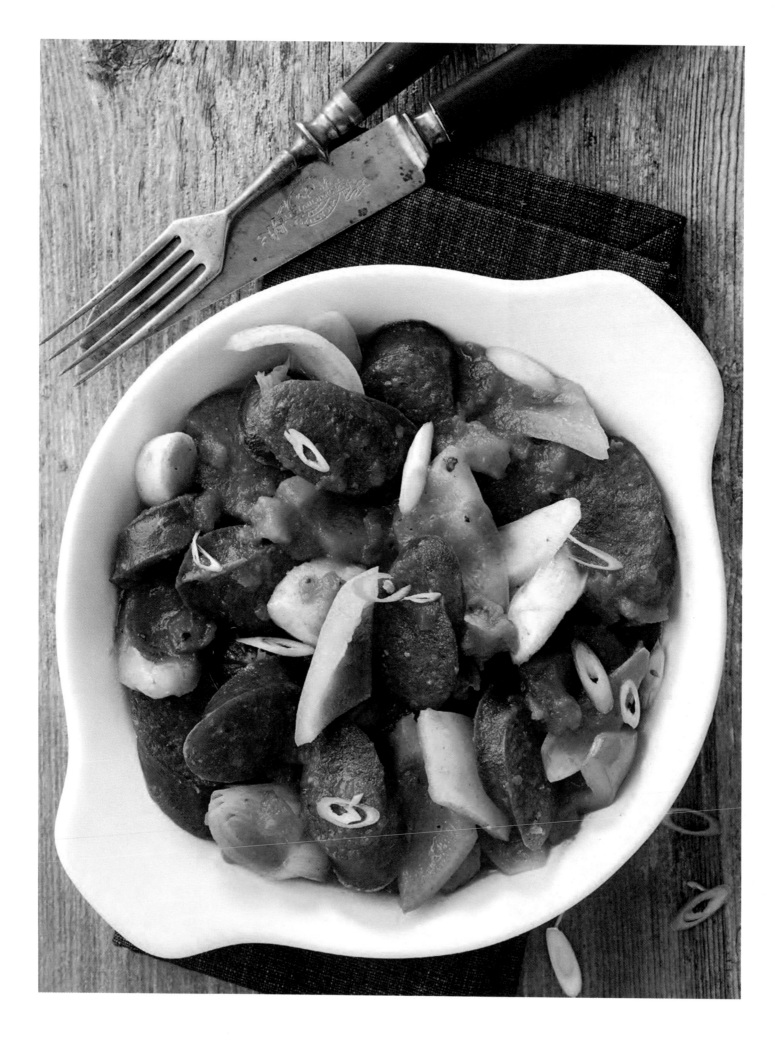

Simple sausage stew

Good sausage is good food. Make sure to pick a sausage that is made from 100 percent meat.

A tasty option is lamb sausage. 10.5 oz (3 hg) of sausage per person, is about enough.
A few tablespoons of butter
1 green bell pepper
1 red bell pepper
1 yellow bell pepper
1 onion
1 small leek
1 can of tomatoes
Broth (optional)
Cayenne pepper

Cut the sausages into rough pieces and sauté in butter for 5 minutes.
Add the bell peppers and roughly chopped onion and sauté a little bit longer. Once everything has a nice color, add the tomatoes and the cayenne pepper. Dilute with broth if necessary and simmer for about 20 minutes.

Perhaps you had a similar sausage stew at school? But then it only tasted of faint sausage, and possibly a little bit of leek. With real sausage as the base, this stew becomes both delicious and healthy. If you eat a normal portion, you'll consume about 800 calories and barely 15 grams of carbohydrates. The fat-burning quotient is 1.5. If you are very weight conscious, you should consume more of the sausage and take down your intake of the vegetables in this dish.

Marianne's Norwegian-style fakir patties

See photo on page 115.

I get so many delicious recipes from my Norwegian pen pals. At first, they were a bit difficult to decipher, but now I know that "tarragon" means "dragon," and "fedd" can refer to a garlic clove. With those descriptions, I was able to decipher the recipe below.

I'm of the opinion that you may as well cook a big batch while you're at it. My Norwegian pen pal seems to be of the same opinion.

1.1 lbs (500 g) ground meat each from chicken, veal, and ox (optional: veal, lamb, elk, etc).
    (So you'll get a total of 3.3 lbs meat)
1.1 lbs (500 g) pure fat (I recommend suet, or lard / SSS).
Mix with plenty of parsley
A lot of garlic (at least 2 cloves, I use about 1.4 oz (40 g) per serving!)
2–3 tablespoons tarragon
2–3 tablespoons oregano
Pepper (a little bit of salt is optional)
Some water is necessary to soften the meat, which gets a very firm texture from the fat.

Blend thoroughly and store in the fridge for 12–24 hours. Shape into hot dogs (fry or grill), patties, or meatballs. Enjoy! I thought they were absolutely delicious!

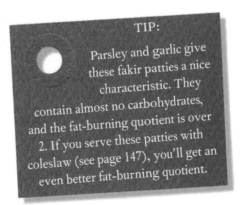

TIP:
Parsley and garlic give these fakir patties a nice characteristic. They contain almost no carbohydrates, and the fat-burning quotient is over 2. If you serve these patties with coleslaw (see page 147), you'll get an even better fat-burning quotient.

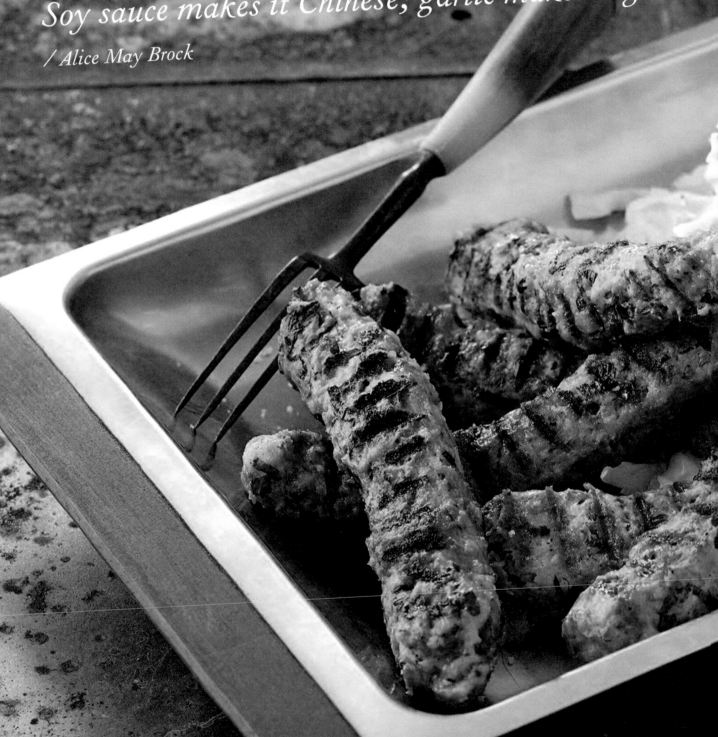

"*Tomatoes and oregano make it Italian; wine and tarragon make it French. Sour cream makes it Russian; lemon and cinnamon make it Greek. Soy sauce makes it Chinese; garlic makes it good.*"

/ Alice May Brock

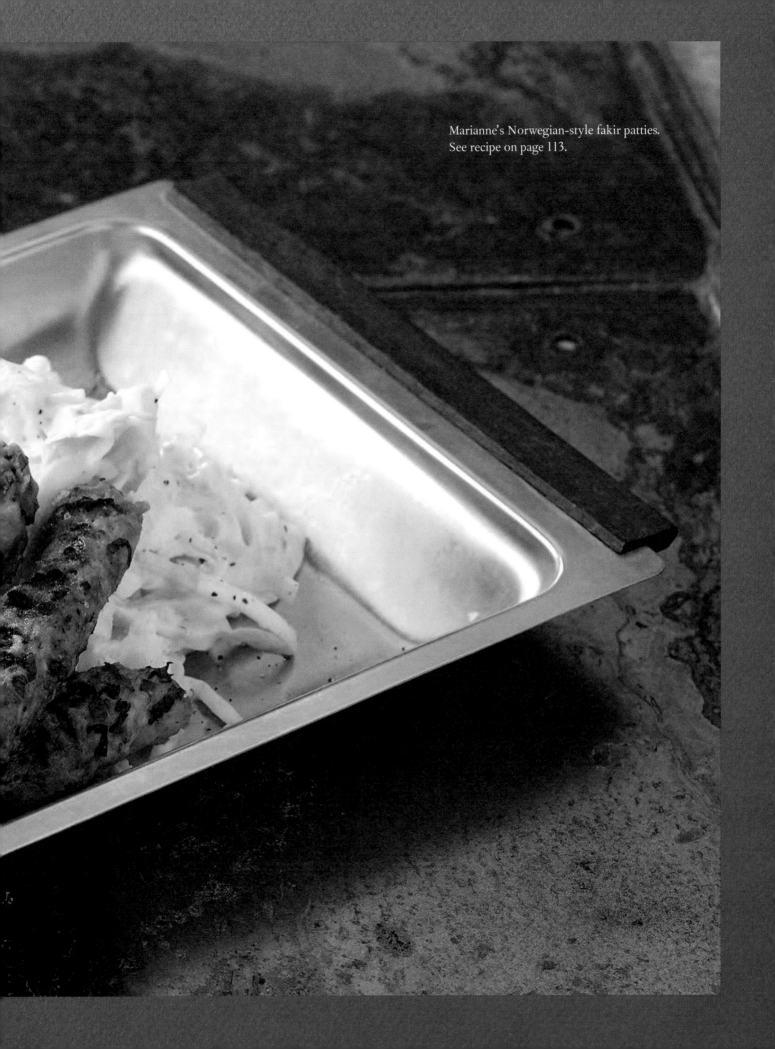

Marianne's Norwegian-style fakir patties.
See recipe on page 113.

A short lesson in meat

Buy meat from animals that have walked freely on green pastures. Make sure that the meat has been tenderized long enough, and that it is at a room temperature when you start cooking it. Those are my most important words of advice.

Meat that contains a lot of marbleized fat is better than lean meat. Meat from cows that have calved a few times is a better option because it has a higher fat content. Meat should always be tenderized well. 60 "degree days" is a good time for tenderization. Degree days is the temperature in Celsius that the meat hangs in, multiplied by the amount of days. If you hang the meat in 5 degrees, you should let it hang for 12 days to achieve 60 degree days. Many grass-fed-meat enthusiasts hang their meat for 70 or 80 degree days.

It can be difficult to find good meat at the grocery store, and most of the time there will be no information available about the tenderization period. Try to find a local farm that raises grass-fed meat and buy your meat from the farm directly.

Vegetables and fish taste the best if they are fresh. Cheese, wine, and meat taste better when aged. When you age meat, it loses water and weighs less. In other words, not very profitable for big meat producers who want to sell as much water as possible to the price of meat. That's why the meat in the store is often not fully tenderized. This is also called vacuum tenderization. Tenderizing meat by hanging it is a far better method, and more expensive. You'll recognize such meat by its darker color, and it usually has a surface that has dried a bit around the edges.

Meat from middle-aged cows is more tender and flavorful than meat from bulls. However, a young, castrated bull may taste just as well. Nice South American meat often comes from steers of Black Angus or Hereford. Meat from animals that are strolling freely on green pastures is always a healthier option because they have a great balance of omega-6 and omega-3 fatty acids. That means that meat is at its best after the animals have spent the summer on green pastures, and at its worst during the winter when the animals are contained in their stalls.

Inexpensive meat usually comes from young bulls that haven't been castrated and have grown too quickly, and their meat is usually not tenderized for very long. The result is boring, tasteless, and lean meat. That's the meat you usually find on sale at your local grocery store. If you want to be cost- and health-conscious when you buy your meat, it is better to choose meat from grass-fed South American animals. These animals don't spend their winters in heated barns where they would have to eat fodder, so therefore their meat is also a better choice for the environment.

Meat that comes from Swedish grass-fed cows that has been tenderized through hanging is of course an excellent choice as well. Cows grow slowly in our climate—a perfect condition for well-marbleized meat. If you buy a large package of meat, you'll get a better pound price—close to the price you would pay at the grocery store for meat of lower quality.

TIP: YOU SHOULD ALWAYS AVOID FAT-FREE FOODS. THEY ARE LEAN AND TASTELESS. THIS IS ESPECIALLY IMPORTANT WHEN IT COMES TO MEAT. IT IS THE FAT IN THE MEAT THAT BRINGS OUT THE FLAVOR.

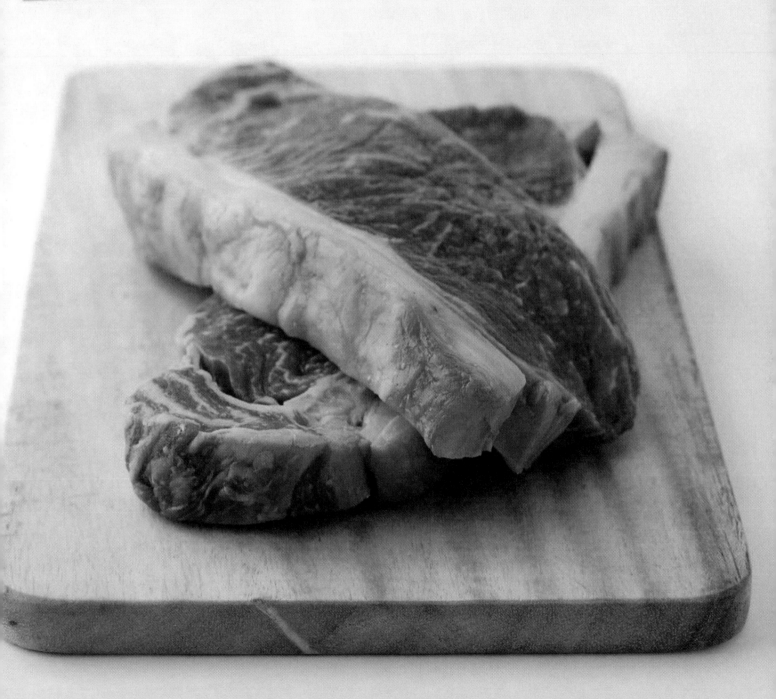

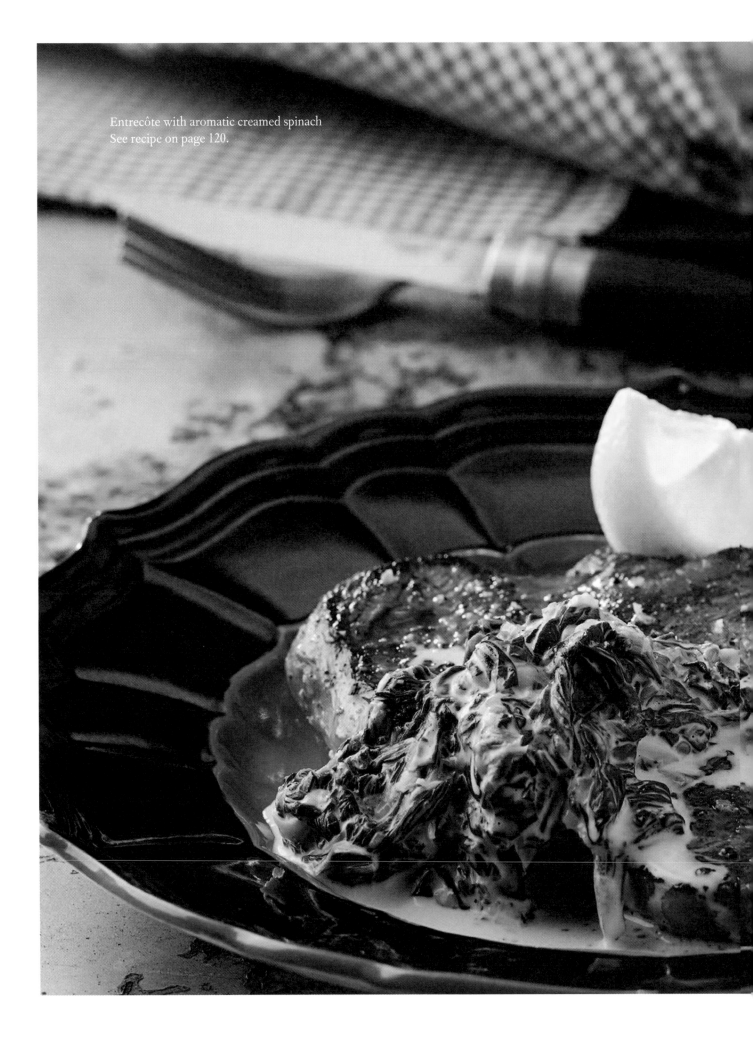

Entrecôte with aromatic creamed spinach
See recipe on page 120.

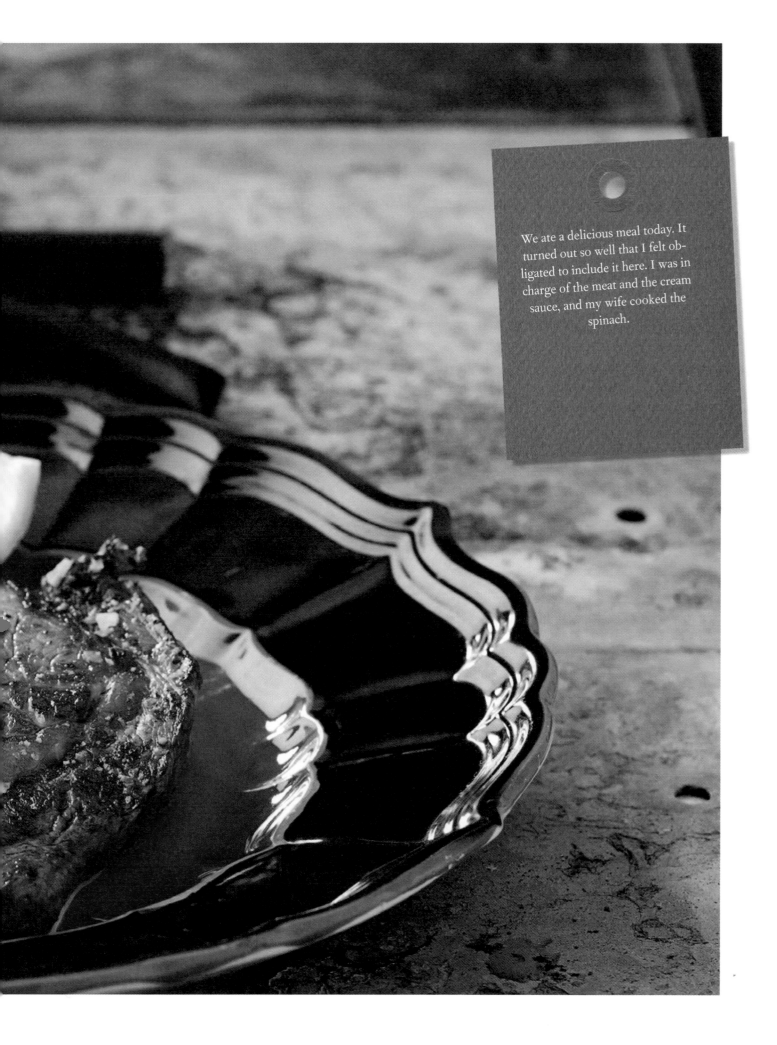

We ate a delicious meal today. It turned out so well that I felt obligated to include it here. I was in charge of the meat and the cream sauce, and my wife cooked the spinach.

Entrecôte with aromatic creamed spinach

See photo on page 118.

2 thick pieces of entrecôte, about 8.8 oz (250 g) each
Salt and coarsely ground black pepper
Butter or oil for sautéing

For the spinach:
14 oz (400 g) spinach
1.8 oz (50 g) butter
Salt and pepper
2 tablespoons *sambal oelek*
⅕ cup (50 g) crème fraiche
⅕ cup (20 g) grated Västerbotten cheese, or Parmesan

For the sauce:
Sliced Parmesan cheese according to your own preference, I used about ⅖ cup (20 g).
⅖–⅘ cup (100–200 ml) heavy whipping cream

Use your hands to flatten the entrecôte steaks. Coat both sides of each piece with salt and plenty of coarsely ground black pepper. Leave the meat alone to acquire room temperature. Thaw and steam off the spinach if it is frozen. Melt the butter and cook the spinach with butter, spices, and *sambal oelek*. Simmer over low heat.

Now it's time to sauté the meat. I use a hot skillet with butter and oil, and I turn the meat once a lot of blood has reached the surface. Once the blood reaches the other side, my meat is cooked. Then the meat has a nice browned surface, but is red inside, and perhaps even a little bit bloody in the middle. If you want your meat more medium cooked, turn it over another time.

Serve the meat on hot plates. Melt sliced Parmesan in the hot skillet and dilute it with cream. While the sauce is cooking (it only takes about a minute), stir crème fraiche and Västerbotten cheese into the spinach. Now that the meat, the sauce, and the creamed spinach are cooked, it is time to serve it all!

A serving of entrecôte with an equal portion of creamed spinach makes for a complete dinner for a person. A meal like that contains about 1,200 calories, 65 grams of protein, and 105 grams of fat. The carbohydrates will vary depending on what sides you serve with this dish, but count on about 7 grams. The fat-burning quotient is about 1.5. Only about 2 percent of the energy comes from carbohydrates, so it is a strict LCHF meal. The nutritional value is extremely good, with more than a whole daily recommendation of a bunch of nutrients. This type of food gives both energy and boosts your health.

Tip: This recipe feeds two hungry people. If you are small in size, it can even feed four people.

Spicy lamb roulade with haricot verts

Lamb and mutton in all shapes and forms are great food options. However, some cuts can be difficult to use. The flank of lamb is one of those cuts, but here is a good solution for that issue.

1 flank of lamb, with or without bone
10.6 oz (300 g) ground lamb
⅕ cup (50 ml) heavy whipping cream
1–2 tablespoons mixed herb spices (thyme, oregano, basil, rosemary)
1 chili, finely chopped
⅕ cup (7 g) parsley, chopped
2 cloves of garlic, finely chopped
1 shallot, finely chopped
1 tablespoon butter
⅖ cup (100 ml) red wine
Salt and pepper

Bone the flank of lamb, or order it boneless from the butcher.

Brown shallot, garlic, and herb spices in butter.

Mix the ground lamb with heavy whipping cream and add all the spices.

Spread the ground mix over the flank of lamb and roll. Secure the roulade with string.

Brown the surface all around the lamb roulade. Transfer it to an ovenproof dish and roast in the oven at 350°F (175°C) for about 40 minutes.

Pour some red wine into the dish towards the end of the cooking time.

Serve with the red wine sauce and haricot verts (see page 145) or coleslaw (see page 147).

The lamb roulade is almost carbohydrate-free, and the fat-burning quotient is above 1. I like to eat this type of meal with coleslaw. A serving of the lamb roulade with coleslaw contains about 700 calories and approximately 5 grams of carbohydrates. The fat-burning quotient is about 1.5.

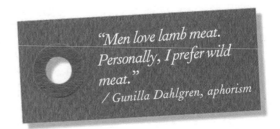

"Men love lamb meat. Personally, I prefer wild meat."
/ Gunilla Dahlgren, aphorism

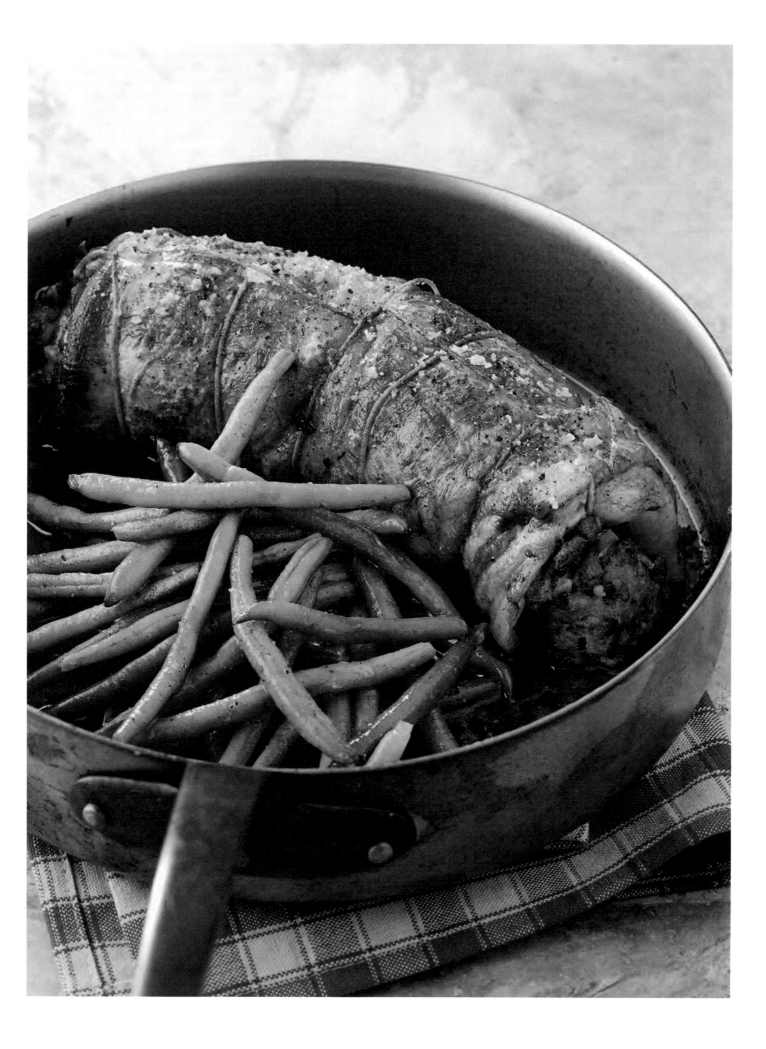

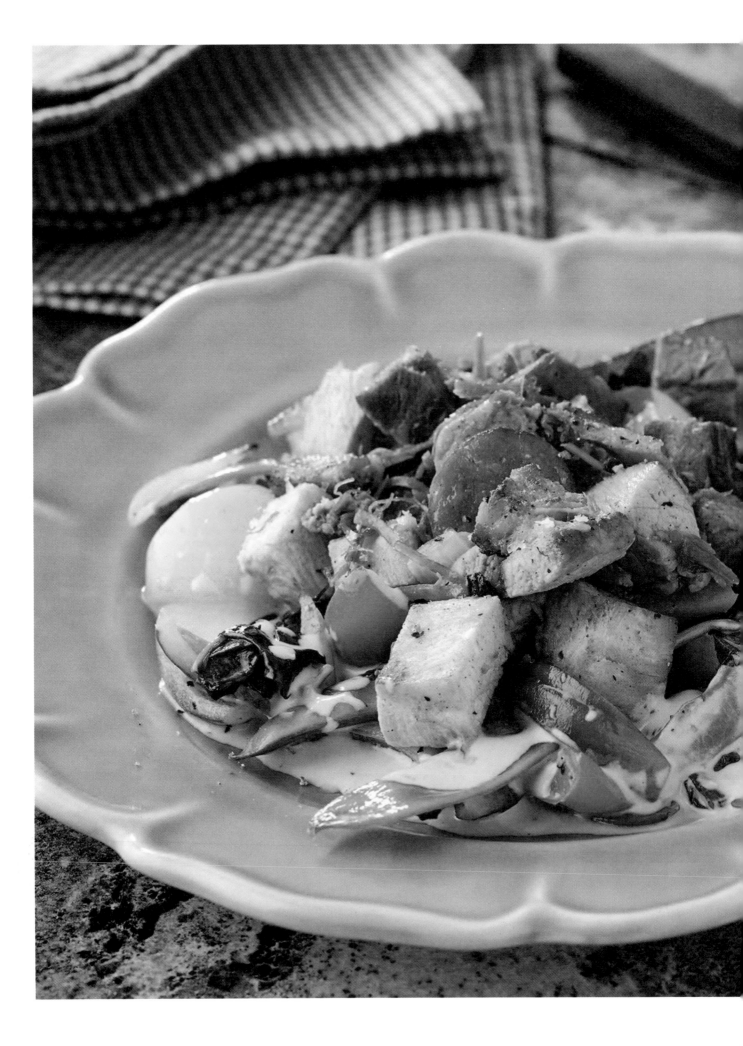

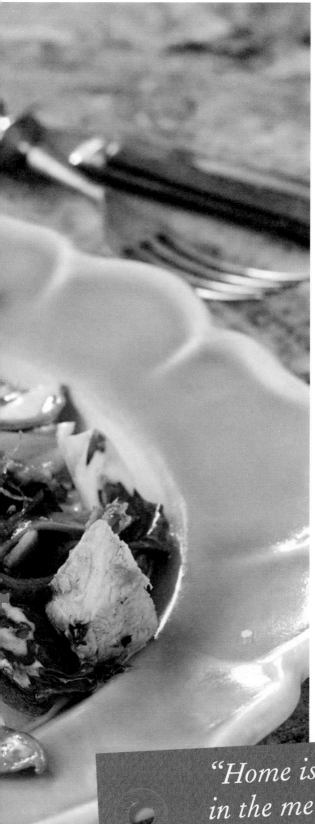

Creamed stir-fry meal for two

10.6–14 oz (3–4 hg) of leftover meat, such as ham, smoke-
  cured loin of pork, chicken, or whatever you may have
1 bag (14 oz/400 g) of mixed vegetables that grow above
  ground, like spinach, pepper, and sugar snap peas
1–2 tablespoons butter
$\frac{2}{5}$ cup (100 ml) heavy whipping cream
Salt and pepper

In a skillet, fry the vegetables in butter, add the cream, and
season.

Chop up your leftover meats and spread them over the
greens.
Serve.

This meal takes about 10 minutes to make. If you have a
little bit more time, you can cook some bacon, keep it warm,
and fry the greens in the bacon fat instead of butter. This
quick dish will then take about 15 minutes to cook from
beginning to end.

If you serve this to two people, you'll get about 8 grams of
carbohydrates per person. The fat-burning quotient is right
below 1.

*"Home is where you know what's
in the meat stew."
/ Danish proverb*

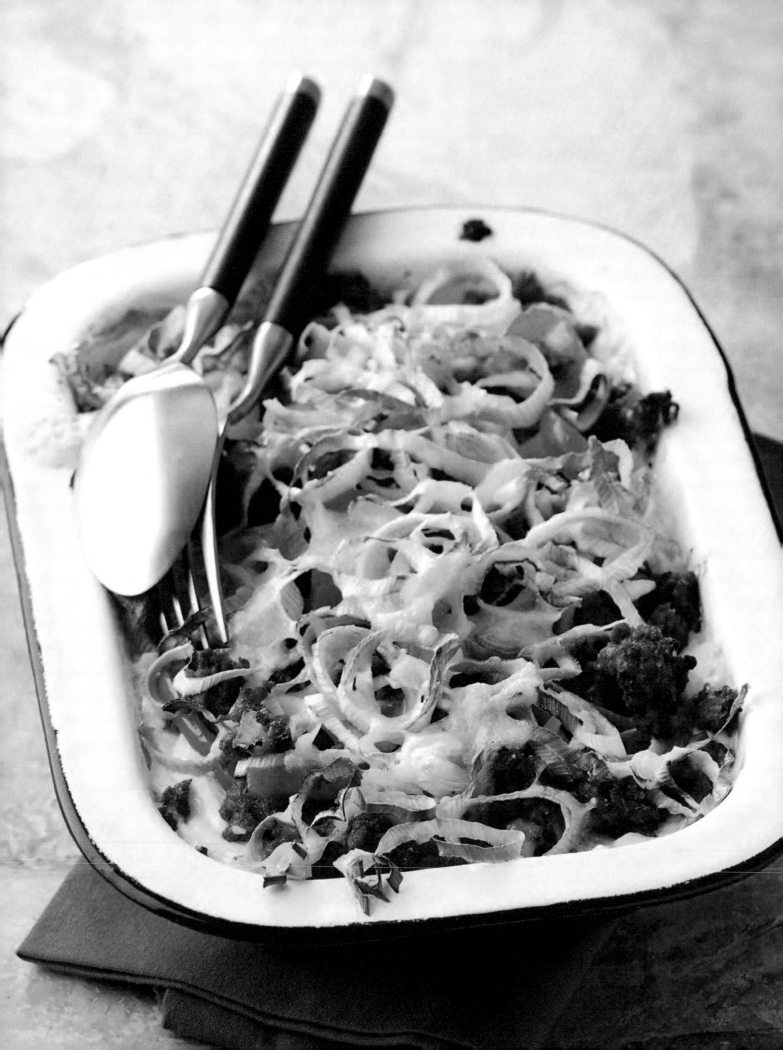

Ingerlise's taco gratin

2.2 lbs (1 kg) mixed ground pork and beef
1–2 yellow onions
1 red bell pepper
1 clove of garlic
4 tablespoons (or 1.4 oz/40 g) taco spice
⅘ cup (150 ml) crushed tomatoes
Salt and pepper
⅘ cup (200 g) crème fraiche
10.6 oz (300 g) cream cheese
Leek
Grated cheese

Preheat the oven to 450°F (225°C).
    Brown the ground meat mix and put it aside. Brown the onion and the bell pepper. Add spices and crushed tomatoes.
    Mix everything with the ground meat.
    Mix cream cheese with crème fraiche and spread the cheese blend in an ovenproof dish.
    Spread the ground meat mix on top. Top the gratin with leek and grated cheese.
    Bake the gratin in the center of the oven for about 15 minutes.

A hearty portion of this gratin contains about 7 grams of carbohydrates and has a fat-burning quotient of about 1.2. Recommended sides: Olive and feta cheese medley (see recipe on page 150).

Lamb in cabbage

See photo on page 126.

I love lamb meat, especially from a full-grown lamb. I also love white cabbage. Combined, they make an excellent cabbage pudding, delicious soups, and lamb in cabbage. Lamb in cabbage is a classic home-cooked meal, and it has the advantage that everything is thrown into the same pot. No need to worry about sides.
    If you have a large pot, you may as well cook ten servings at once. It is no more work than cooking one dinner. My variation of this dish contains about double the amount of meat as cabbage. We want our food to be as healthy as possible.

At least 2.2 lbs (1 kg) lamb meat, breast or shoulder cut is
    good
1.1 lbs (500 g) white cabbage
Plenty of butter for sautéing, I use about 3.5 oz
Salt, white peppercorns, bay leaves, water
Bouillon cube (optional)

I take out the big cast iron pot and begin by browning coarsely chopped meat. The remaining meat, I sauté in rounds in one or two skillets. (If I throw all the meat into the pot at once, it will boil rather than brown.)
    Once I've browned all the meat and put it in the pot, I add some water to the skillets, whisk, and add that liquid to the pot. I season with 10–20 white peppercorns and at least half a tablespoon of salt. One or two bay leaves are added as well, and a bouillon cube if I feel like it.
    Then I cover the pot with a lid, and leave it on very low heat. Leave it like that for a while.
    One hour prior to serving the dish, I add coarsely chopped white cabbage to the pot and add some more liquid. Once the cabbage has softened, the meal is ready. Garnish with some chopped parsley to make it look extra nice.

If you use the double amount of meat as white cabbage, the fat-burning quotient per serving will be about 1.3, and the meal will have 500 calories and about 3.5 grams of carbohydrates.

Lamb in cabbage
See recipe on page 125.

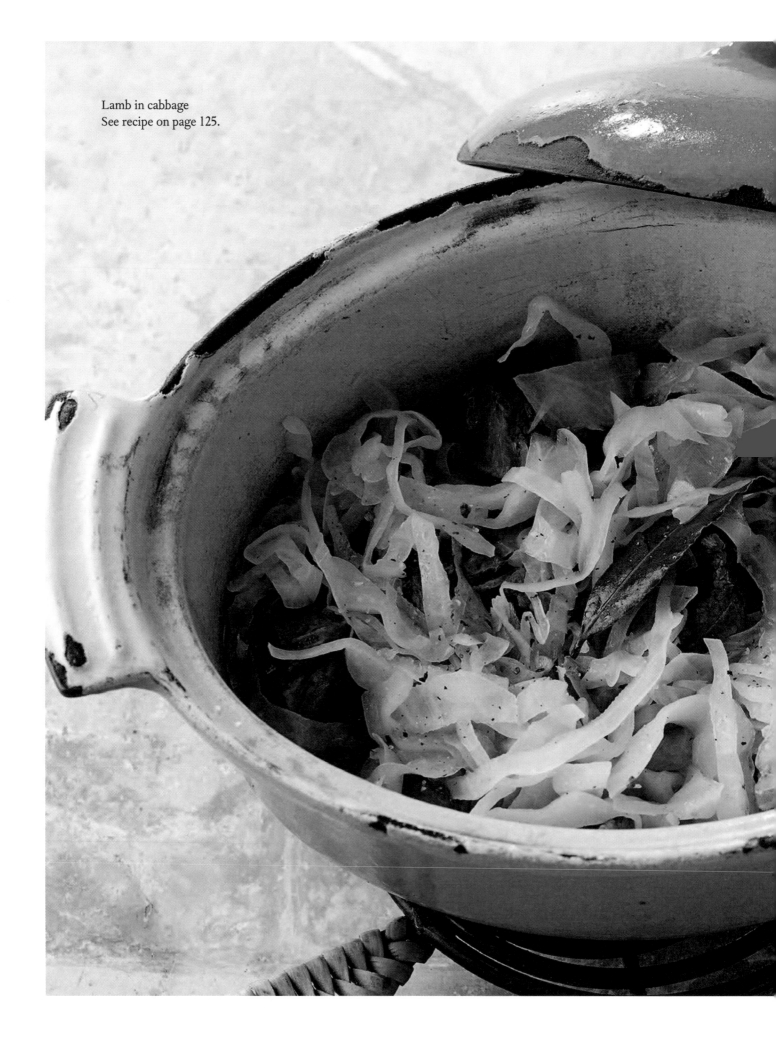

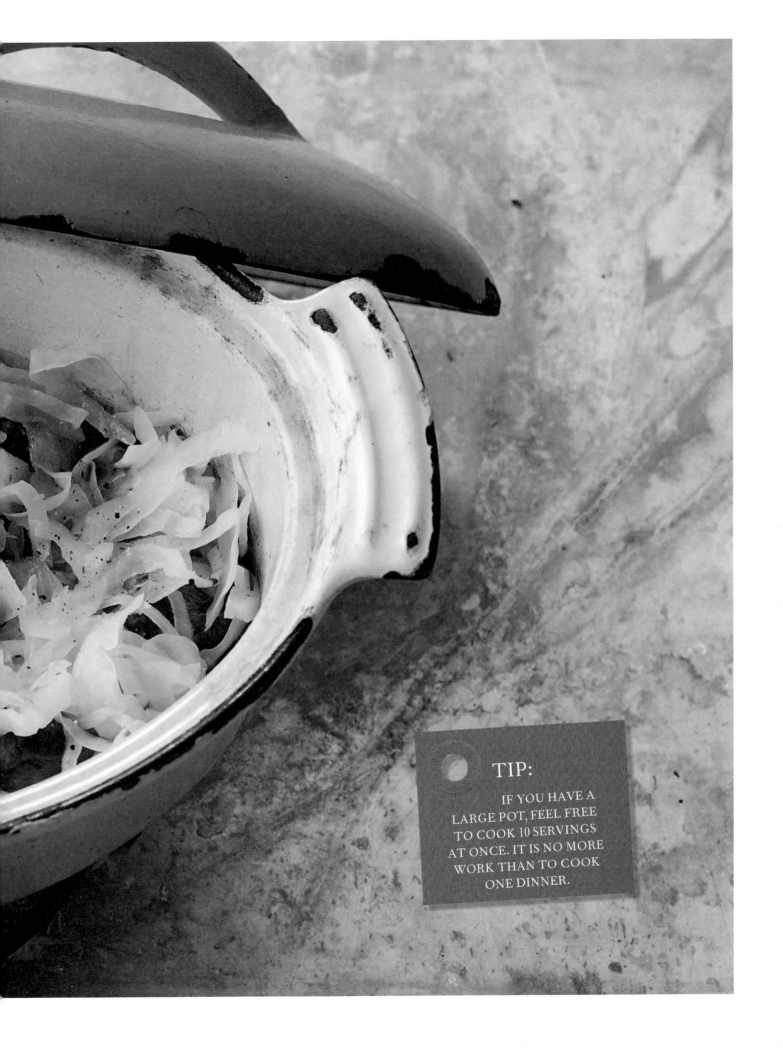

TIP:

IF YOU HAVE A
LARGE POT, FEEL FREE
TO COOK 10 SERVINGS
AT ONCE. IT IS NO MORE
WORK THAN TO COOK
ONE DINNER.

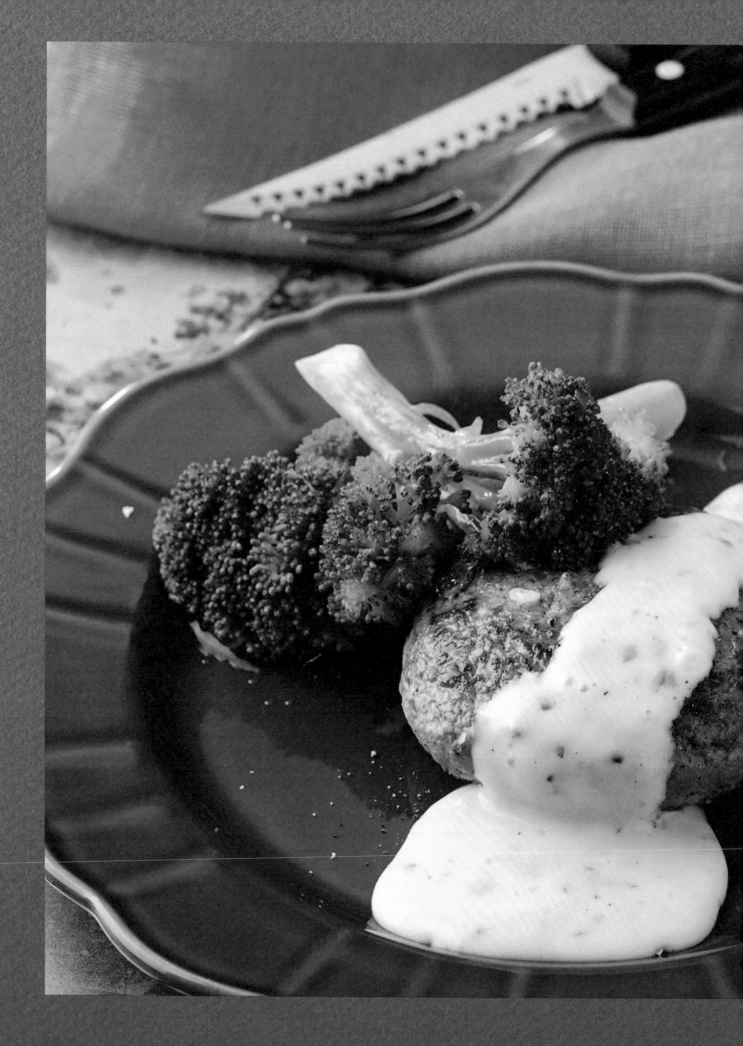

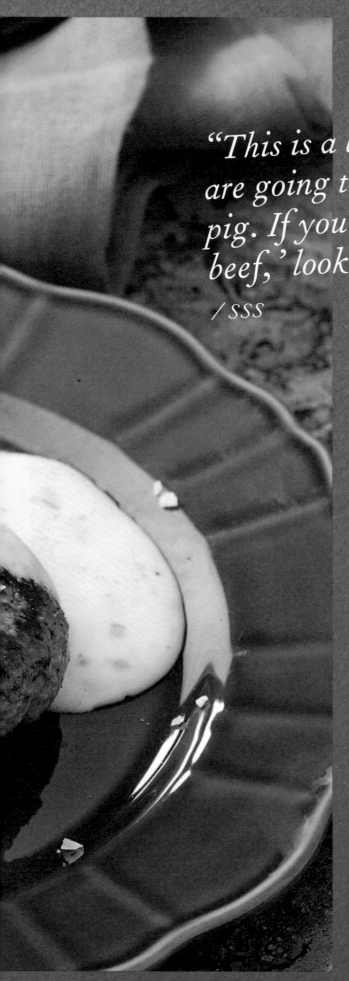

"This is a book about real food. If you are going to cook a pork chop, look for a pig. If you are going to make a 'sailor's beef,' look for a sailor."

/ SSS

Quick ground beef patties with even quicker béarnaise

1.3–1.75 lbs (600–800 g) ground beef
2 tablespoons butter for sautéing
1 teaspoon salt
Coarsely ground black pepper

Shape four beef patties out of the ground beef and season the surfaces with salt and pepper.

Sauté in butter until the patties have a nice color.

Bring all the ingredients for the quick béarnaise sauce to a boil (see recipe on page 159).

Serve with any vegetable of your choice (that grows above ground), or with a green salad (recipe on page 39).

One beef patty with sauce provides about 700 calories, but only contains about 2 grams of carbohydrates. The fat-burning quotient is about 1.5. Great diet food! One serving of butter cooked broccoli adds about 2 grams of carbohydrates.

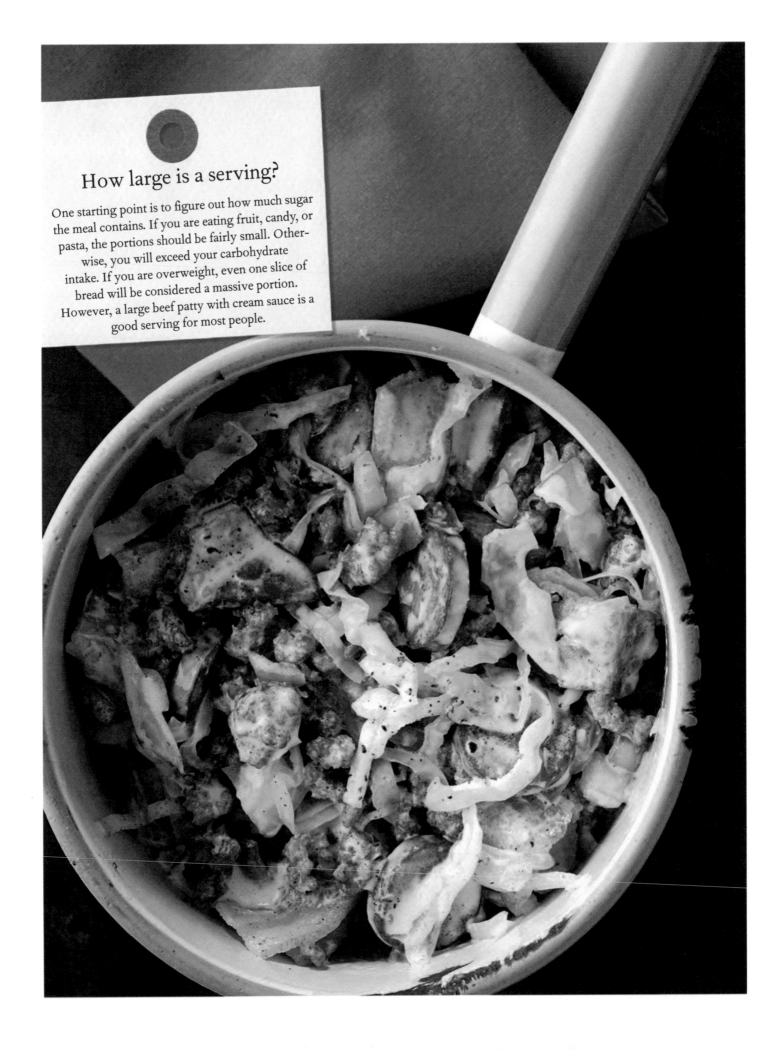

How large is a serving?

One starting point is to figure out how much sugar the meal contains. If you are eating fruit, candy, or pasta, the portions should be fairly small. Otherwise, you will exceed your carbohydrate intake. If you are overweight, even one slice of bread will be considered a massive portion. However, a large beef patty with cream sauce is a good serving for most people.

Sörmland box

Bigos is a type of sauerkraut stew with sausage and pork. It is often described as the national dish of Poland. One of my Swedish pen pals, signed MiaP, has created a variation that is delicious, filling, and healthy.

1.1 lbs (500 g) ground meat, preferably a mix of pork and beef, or just pork
1 package of bacon
1–2 yellow onions
2–3 spicy sausages, such as Chorizo
½ small head of white cabbage (or equal amount of sauerkraut)
Pepper, preferably a variety of different kinds
2 teaspoons soy sauce
⅖ cup (100 ml) heavy whipping cream
⅖ cup (100 ml) crème fraiche

Fry bacon and chopped yellow onion for a few minutes. Pour into a roasting pot.
Sauté the ground meat in the bacon fat and butter. Then add it to the roasting pot.
Sauté the sliced sausages and add to the pot.
Add the shredded cabbage. Season with soy sauce and pepper; salt won't be necessary.
Add heavy whipping cream and crème fraiche and simmer over low heat for about 15 minutes.
Serve on warm plates, and garnish with something green.

One serving of this rich and hearty meal contains about 600–700 calories and approximately 5–8 grams of carbohydrates, depending on the kind of cabbage you are using. Sauerkraut contains fewer carbohydrates than white cabbage. The fat-burning quotient is above 1. If you make this stew with sauerkraut, ground pork, and fatty sausage of the ethnic variety, you'll even be able to achieve a fat-burning quotient of 2.

Hash

See photo on page 132.

Let's say your fridge is packed with leftovers, but you don't feel like eating them cold. Well, then you could chop up some meats and sauté them with onion. I made chopped saddle of lamb and onion, a little bit of ham steak, and a fried egg. Traditional hash contains potatoes, but we are leaving them out.

You can use leftovers from any meats for this dish. Roast beef is a classic. You can also use lamb steak, ham steak, meat-packed sausage, chicken, salmon, or whatever you may have at hand. Try using two or three kinds. It will all marry nicely in the pan!
Onion is absolutely necessary, yellow or red
Egg
Extra sides are optional. Try fried halloumi, or mushrooms.
Fat for sautéing, I use butter and oil
Salt and pepper

Suggested sides:
French mustard
HP sauce, or Worcestershire sauce
Pickles (salty)
Capers and/or pickled beets (Watch the carbohydrates!)

Chop the onion and sauté until it has a shiny surface. If the remaining ingredients are cooked already, chop them up and add to the onion and heat up. Otherwise, sauté the meats. Add salt and pepper. I tend to fry the eggs in a separate skillet, but if you don't care, you can just push the "hash" aside, and fry the egg in the same skillet. You also have the option to serve the egg yolk raw in half an eggshell.

The nutritional value of this type of hash depends on what you use when making it. Today, my hash contained about 7 oz (200 g) meat and about 7 oz (200 g) of the remaining ingredients. That provided me with about 700 calories, 55 grams of protein, 53 grams of fat, and 7 grams of carbohydrates. That's a little more protein than I normally eat in one sitting, but it was delicious. Four percent of the energy content comes from carbohydrates, so it is an LCHF-diet-approved meal. You'll get the fat-burning quotient by dividing the fat weight (53 grams) by the remaining ingredients (55 g + 7 g). That gives us 0.85, which is pretty decent. If you want to improve the fat value, get rid of the egg white and add a dollop of butter. Then you'll get up to a fat-burning quotient of 1.

Hash
See recipe on page 131.

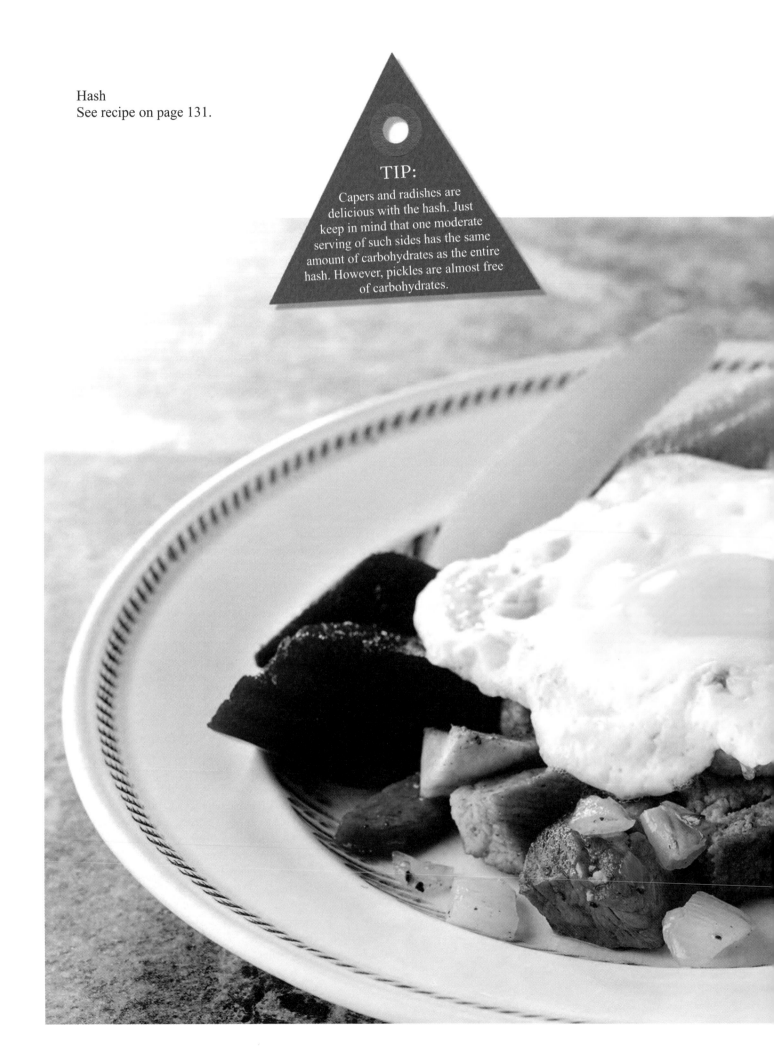

TIP:
Capers and radishes are delicious with the hash. Just keep in mind that one moderate serving of such sides has the same amount of carbohydrates as the entire hash. However, pickles are almost free of carbohydrates.

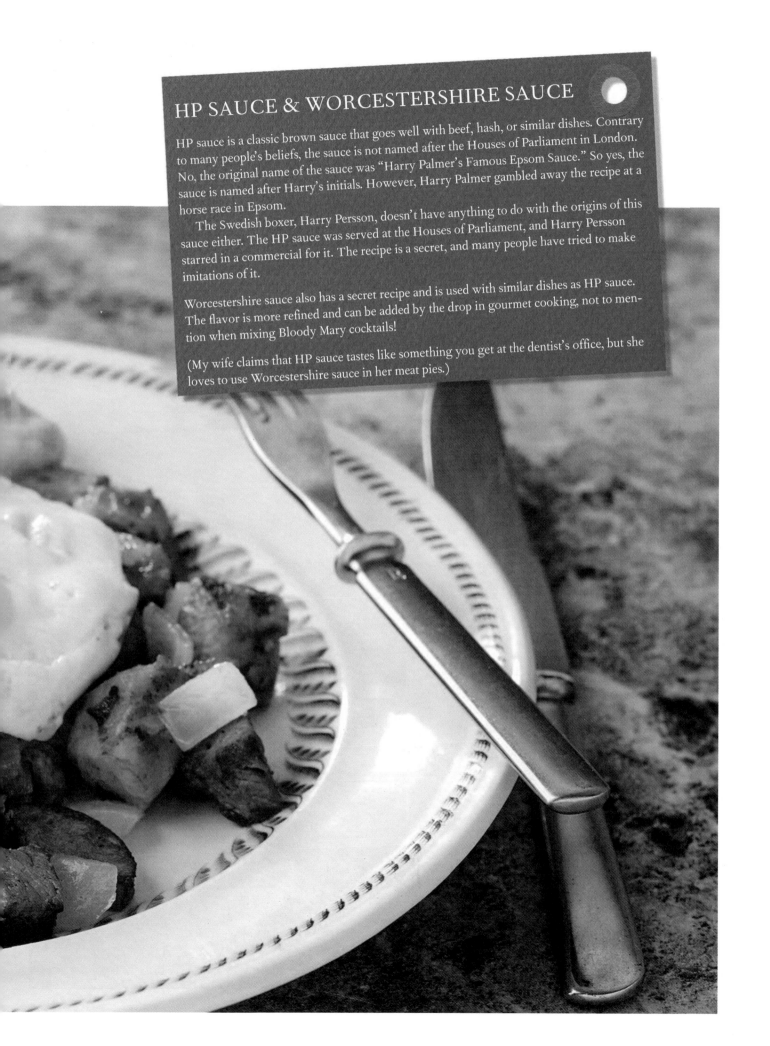

HP SAUCE & WORCESTERSHIRE SAUCE

HP sauce is a classic brown sauce that goes well with beef, hash, or similar dishes. Contrary to many people's beliefs, the sauce is not named after the Houses of Parliament in London. No, the original name of the sauce was "Harry Palmer's Famous Epsom Sauce." So yes, the sauce is named after Harry's initials. However, Harry Palmer gambled away the recipe at a horse race in Epsom.

The Swedish boxer, Harry Persson, doesn't have anything to do with the origins of this sauce either. The HP sauce was served at the Houses of Parliament, and Harry Persson starred in a commercial for it. The recipe is a secret, and many people have tried to make imitations of it.

Worcestershire sauce also has a secret recipe and is used with similar dishes as HP sauce. The flavor is more refined and can be added by the drop in gourmet cooking, not to mention when mixing Bloody Mary cocktails!

(My wife claims that HP sauce tastes like something you get at the dentist's office, but she loves to use Worcestershire sauce in her meat pies.)

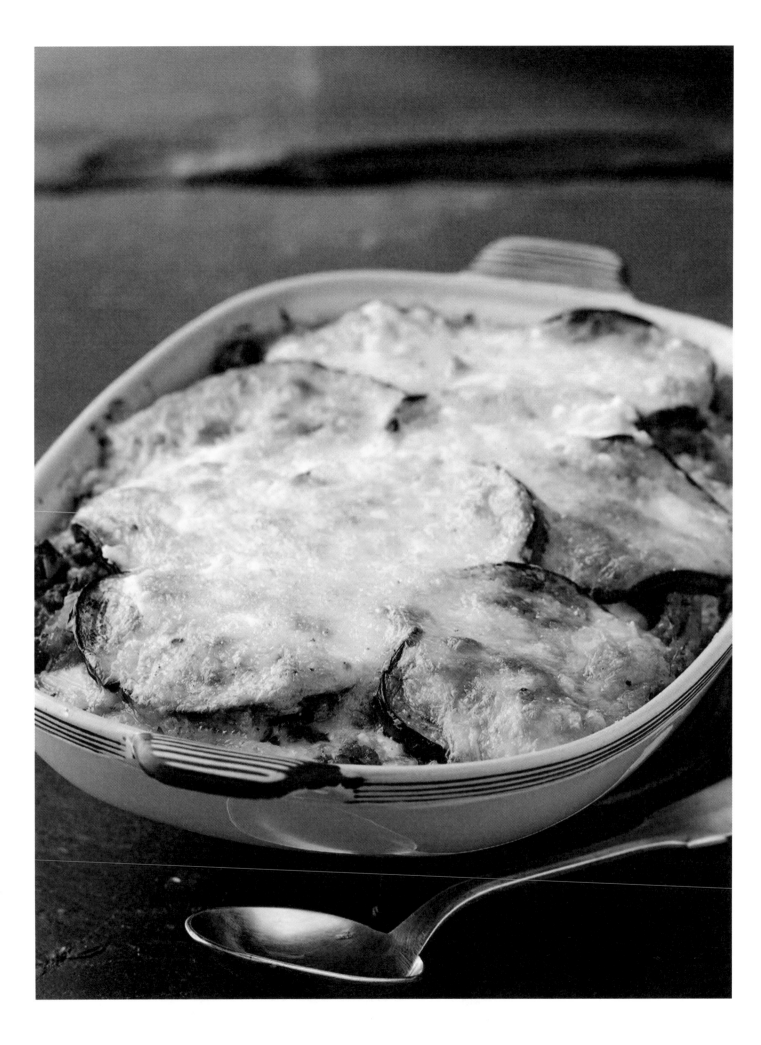

Moussaka

Moussaka consists of eggplant, ground meat sauce, and cheese sauce in a gratin. Let's call it Greek lasagna. However, it is way healthier and contains a lot fewer carbohydrates than its Italian counterpart.

2 eggplants, sliced
1 tablespoon butter
1 tablespoon olive oil

For the meat sauce:
1.1–1.3 lbs (500–600 g) ground beef, or ground lamb
1 tablespoon butter and/or olive oil
2 yellow onions, chopped
1–3 garlic cloves, according to your own preference
½ teaspoon *sambal oelek*, or any other chili
1 teaspoon cumin
1 tablespoon oregano
1–2 teaspoons paprika
Powdered bouillon or fond to get enough salt (salt if necessary)
3 tablespoons tomato purée
⅖–⅘ cup (100–200 ml) water

For the cheese sauce:
⅘ cup (200 ml) heavy whipping cream
⅘ cup (80 g) grated whole milk cheese
⅕ cup (20 g) Parmesan
Salt, white pepper, nutmeg
3 egg yolks

Slice the eggplant and sauté the slices in oil/butter. Add salt and pepper. Set aside.

Sauté the ground meat, add the remaining ingredients, and simmer the sauce until it thickens.

Bring the cream for the cheese sauce to a boil, set the pot aside, and stir in cheese and spices. Allow the sauce to cool a bit before you mix in the egg yolks.

Layer eggplant slices with meat sauce in an ovenproof dish and pour the cheese sauce on top. Up to this point, you can prepare the dish in advance. Bake in the oven at 350°F (175°C) for 20–30 minutes.

Serve with tzatziki (see page 150).

This moussaka portion is enough to fill four fairly hungry bellies. Each serving contains about 750 calories and 8–9 grams of carbohydrates. The fat-burning quotient is 1.3. The tzatziki adds about 4 carbohydrates per serving.

Beef stroganoff

According to legend, the Russian count, Alexander Sergejevitj Stroganoff, was toothless. Therefore, his personal chef needed to create dishes that could be swallowed without having to chew them first. Beef stroganoff is one of those dishes, and surely it melts in the mouth. The basic idea behind this course is to cook tender meat and mushrooms in soured cream. Onion, tomato purée, and paprika are commonly used to flavor this dish.

When I make stroganoff, I start out with beef from an animal that has been grass-fed. Argentina, Uruguay, New Zealand, and Ireland usually produce price-worthy, high-quality meat. Despite the long time of transport, it is still a better choice for the environment than to buy domestic, industrial-produced meat at the grocery store.

There are sugar-free tomato purée options; always choose those brands before purées with added sugar. Then you'll save yourself the extra carbohydrates. This recipe is intended for six people.

2.2 lbs (1 kg) tender beef
2 medium-size onions
7 oz (200 g) fresh mushrooms
1¾ cups (400 ml) heavy whipping cream
1 jar crème fraiche (7 oz/200 g)
3–4 tablespoons sugar-free tomato purée
1 tablespoon Dijon mustard
⅖–⅘ cup (100–200 ml) white wine, or 1 tablespoon lemon juice
Salt and black pepper. Paprika if you'd like.
Butter for sautéing.

Chop a pair of medium-size onions and carefully sauté in a couple tablespoons butter. The onion should get a shiny surface. Remove the onion and set aside when it is done. If you want fewer carbohydrates, dispose of half the onion after you sauté it; the flavor will remain in the skillet.

Add more butter, increase the heat, and brown the beef (slice it first) with the mushrooms. You may need to sauté them in several rounds to get a nice brown surface.

Mix everything together in the skillet, or in a pot. Season with salt and pepper.

Add the heavy whipping cream and stir. Then you can flavor the stew with the remaining ingredients.

Cover with a lid and boil until the meat is tender. If you serve this dish on a few leafy greens, you'll get about 700 calories, and 6–7 grams of carbohydrates per serving.

The fat-burning quotient is about 1.5. If you want to decrease your carbohydrate intake, first and foremost decrease the amount of onions that you add, then the lemon juice, and the tomato purée. However, if you get below 4 carbohydrates per serving, you'll start to lose the characteristics of this dish.

Beef stroganoff
See recipe on page 135.

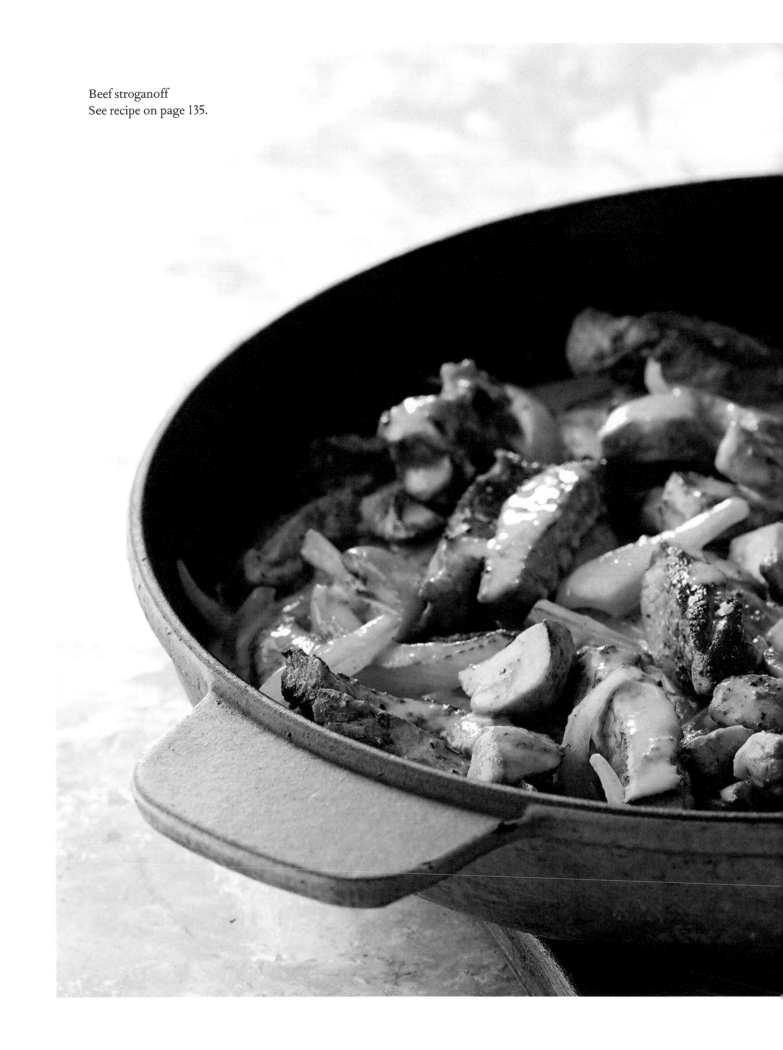

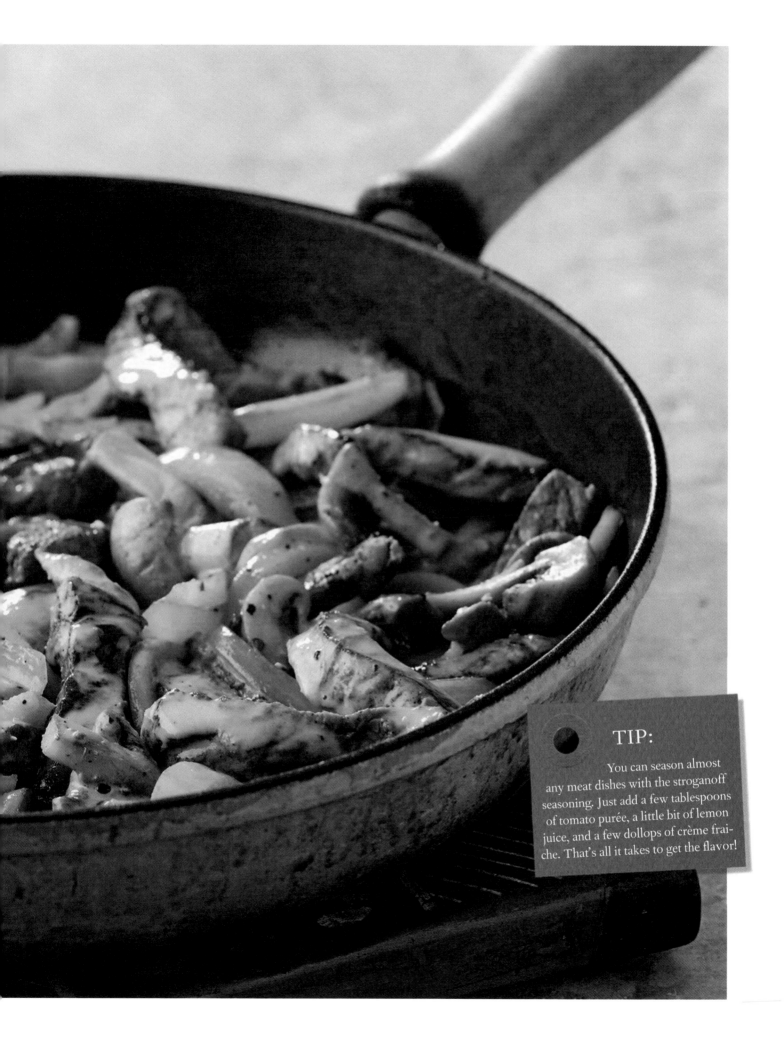

TIP:

You can season almost any meat dishes with the stroganoff seasoning. Just add a few tablespoons of tomato purée, a little bit of lemon juice, and a few dollops of crème fraiche. That's all it takes to get the flavor!

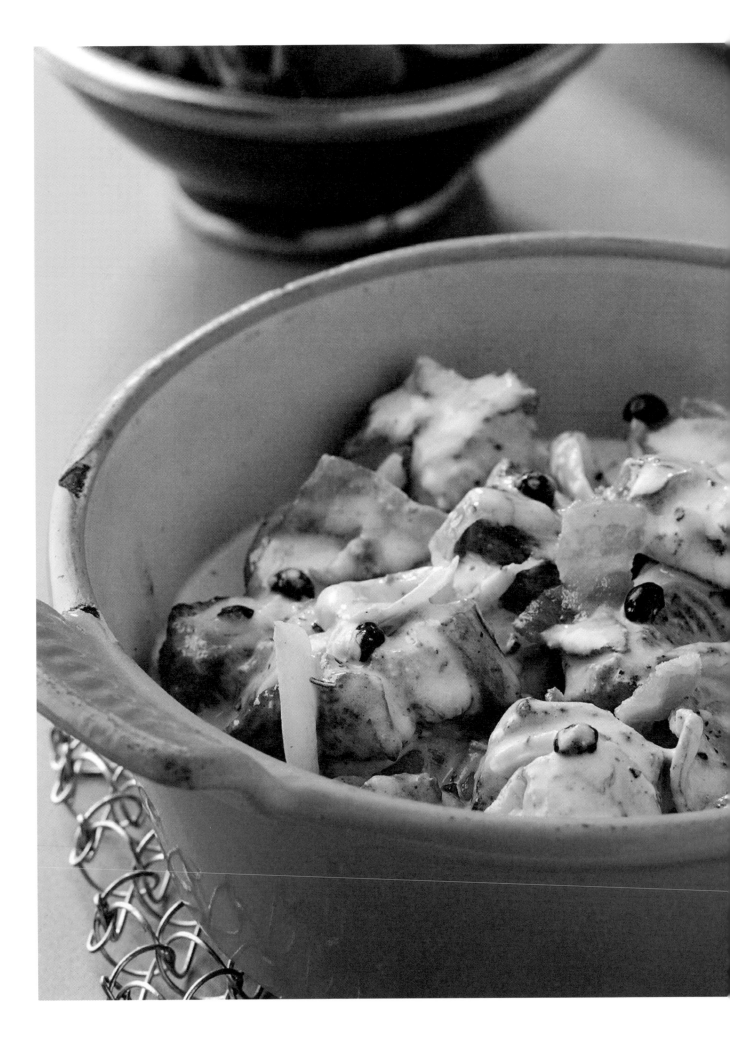

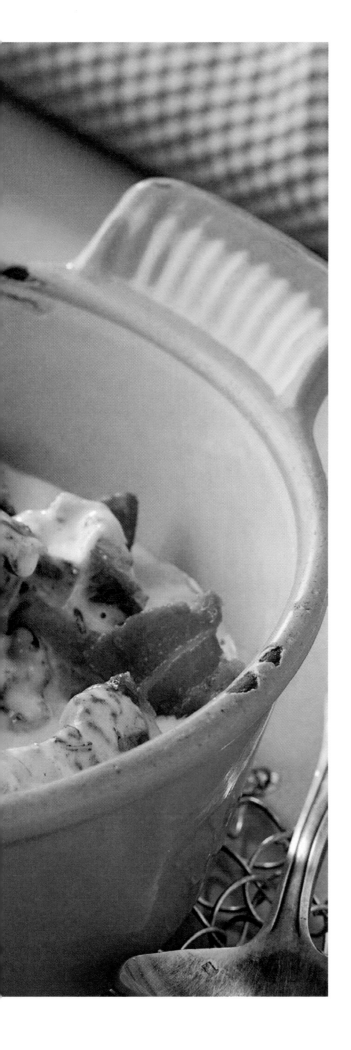

Super simple game stew

Game meat is delicious but very lean. If you sauté game, serve it with a high-fat sauce. If you boil it, add some cream. Then you'll improve the nutritional value and the energy content. Making a stew out of game is perhaps the easiest type of cooking you'll ever do. The only trick is to find the appropriate wine that goes with it!

Any type of game meat, cut into medium-sized pieces
One small onion per person
Crème fraiche/cream
Butter/olive oil for sautéing
Salt, pepper, and soy sauce for flavor
Juniper berries/rosemary, if you want to enhance the
    game flavor.

Brown the meat and add the onions. If you are sautéing a lot of meat, you should do it in rounds, so that you don't get too much liquid in the skillet.
    Dilute with crème fraiche/cream until you have a good consistency.
    Add the spices and boil

Recommended sides: Green salad (recipe on page 39).

A good-size portion of this dish contains about 6 grams of carbohydrates. The fat-burning quotient is about 1.

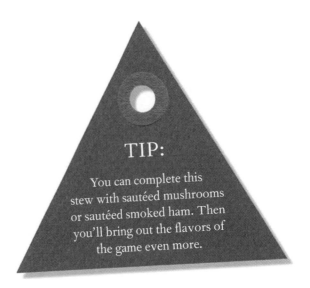

TIP:
You can complete this stew with sautéed mushrooms or sautéed smoked ham. Then you'll bring out the flavors of the game even more.

A few words about lamb

Lamb and sheep meat are among some of the healthiest things we can consume. The reason is simple. These delicious animals usually get to roam freely on green pastures. Which means that they taste the way they were intended to, and that their meat and offal have the nutritional value that nature intended. Personally, I buy my lamb meat from local farms.

We should only eat meat from grass-fed lambs. That may sound obvious to you, but some farmers treat their lambs the way they treat caged hens, or pigs and cows that are contained in stalls way too small for their sizes. Those are the farmers we want to boycott. It would be a disaster if natural lamb meat became as rare as natural pork. So far we have good availability of locally produced, organic lamb meat.

Grass-fed lamb meat is a must in other words, and naturally the meat should be from meat farmers, and not wool producers. Because lamb isn't consumed as much as other meats, industrialization of lamb meat production hasn't developed as vastly as other meat production. Most lamb farmers are still small-scale businesses, with perhaps a dozen ewes in their stable. Seek out a farmer like that and order your lamb meat and lamb liver from them directly. Then you'll get locally produced and slaughtered meat for a great price.

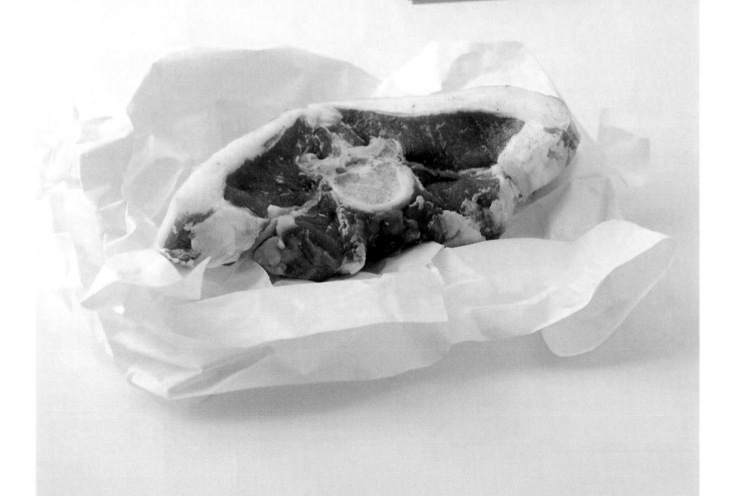

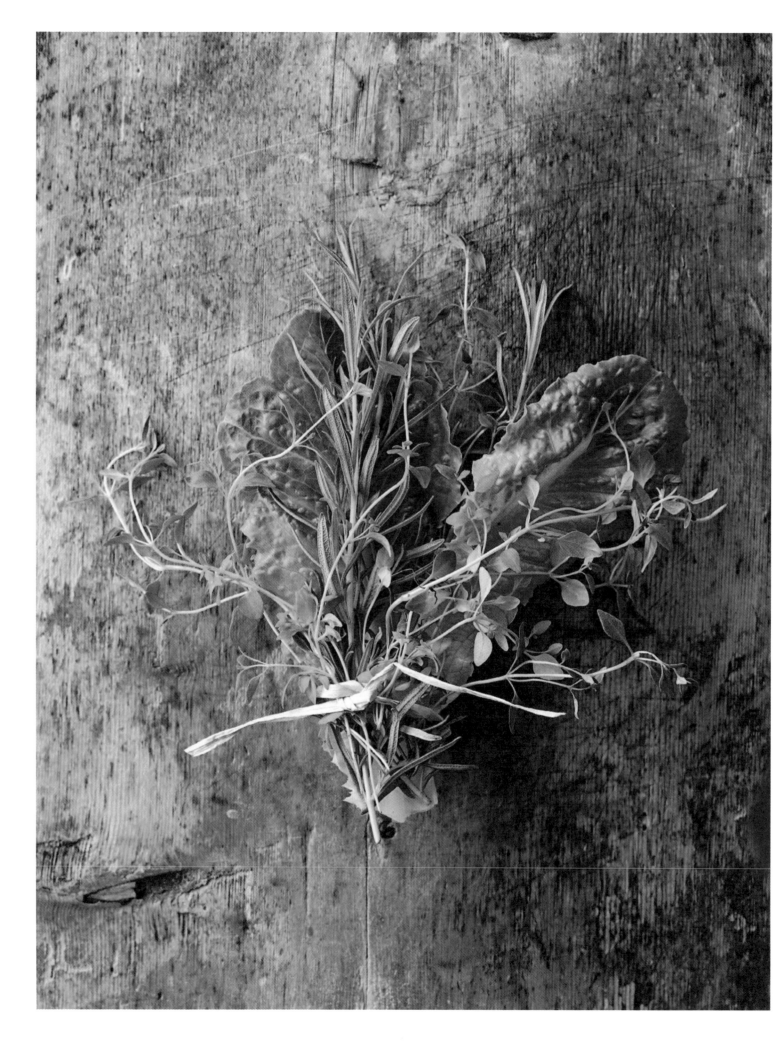

Sides & Condiments

Sauces, breads, dressings, dips, and other delicious condiments

6.

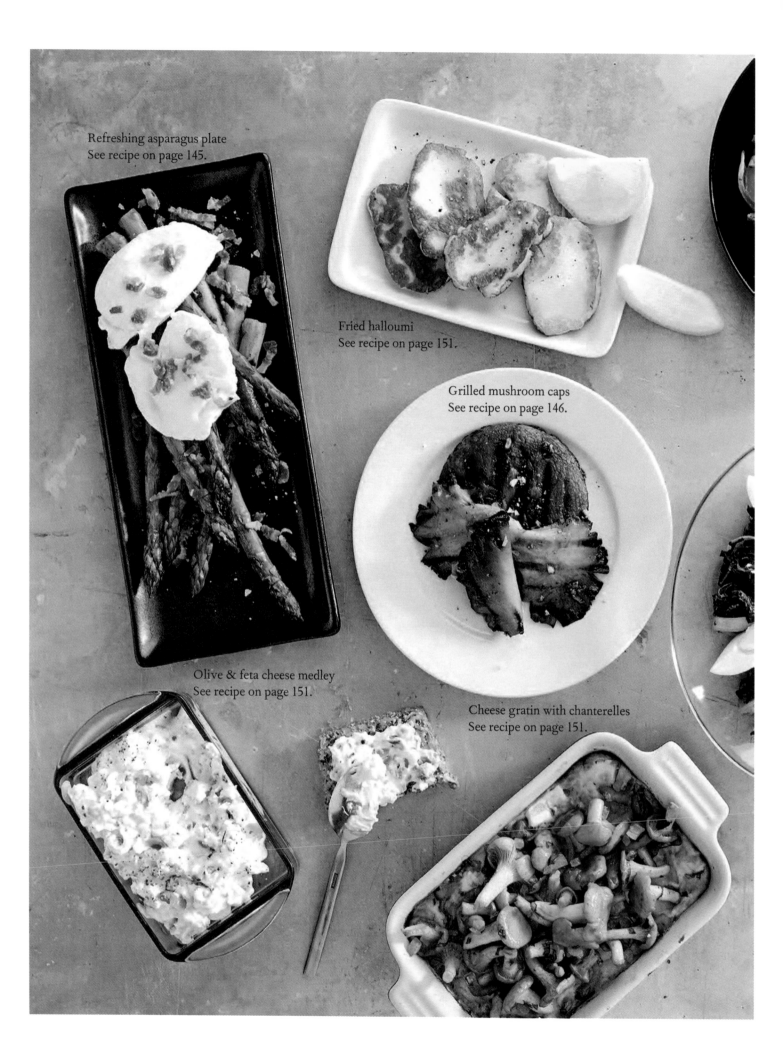

Refreshing asparagus plate
See recipe on page 145.

Fried halloumi
See recipe on page 151.

Grilled mushroom caps
See recipe on page 146.

Olive & feta cheese medley
See recipe on page 151.

Cheese gratin with chanterelles
See recipe on page 151.

Delicious sides
Refreshing asparagus plate

This recipe is super-easy, and the meal is delicious!

Eggs, 1–2 per person

Crispy bacon, about half a pack per person

Asparagus, I prefer green

Butter

One lemon

Salt and pepper

A few green leaves (optional)

Begin by poaching the eggs, if you can. It looks really nice on the plate. However, if you haven't mastered poaching, soft boiled eggs will do just fine.

Cook the bacon until crispy.

Sauté asparagus in butter and bacon fat (or grill it).

Melt some extra butter and flavor with lemon zest and some fresh lemon juice.

Serve leafy greens and asparagus on a plate, then the eggs, and top it off with some finely chopped bacon. Pour the melted lemon butter over and sprinkle with some salt flakes and black pepper. Done!

This is a side that is as delicious as it is easy to make, but the nutritional value is through the roof. With two eggs per person, you'll get about 4 grams of carbohydrates and a fat-burning quotient of 1.5. Count on about 500 calories per serving.

Creamed spinach

Sauté 14 oz (400 g) of spinach in butter, and add ⅘ cup (200 ml) heavy whipping cream into the spinach, cooking for a bit. Season according to your own taste. Some walnuts gives the spinach a nice crispy contrast.

Creamed spinach is a tasty and mild side that goes well with any type of meat.

Green gentlemen in envelopes

Haricot verts are string beans that have been harvested early. They are a classic side for any meat dish, but also taste great in a salad.

Haricot verts

Garlic

Yellow onion

French dressing

Salt and pepper

Butter for sautéing

Quickly sauté the haricot verts in butter.

Season with salt and pepper. Sprinkle with a pressed garlic clove.

Transfer to a bowl and allow to cool.

Add a little bit of finely chopped onion, and French dressing.

A small serving contains about 200 calories and 3 grams of carbohydrates. The fat-burning quotient is about 5.

Spinach with onion

Spinach and onion make a lovely marriage. Use about 4 parts spinach for one part onion and you'll achieve a nice consistency and a moderate amount of carbohydrates.

One bag of parboiled spinach (1.3 lbs/600 g)

2 large onions

1 garlic clove (optional)

4–5 tablespoons butter

½ lemon

Salt and pepper

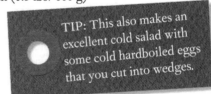

TIP: This also makes an excellent cold salad with some cold hardboiled eggs that you cut into wedges.

Sauté the coarsely chopped onions in butter until they get a shiny surface.

Add the spinach. Boil over moderate heat.

Season with the juice of half a lemon, salt, and pepper. Add some pressed garlic if you like.

One serving (about 7 oz/200 g) provides 140 calories and about 4 grams of carbohydrates. If you want fewer carbohydrates, remove the onion. The fat-burning quotient is about 1.5 if you follow this recipe. You can easily raise it to 3 by adding cream or crème fraiche.

Grilled mushroom caps

If you're lucky, you'll find really large and beautiful mushroom caps out in nature. Some varieties with gorgeous caps include the penny buns and the parasol mushrooms. White mushrooms are fine too, just make sure that whoever is picking them really knows what they are doing. The parasol mushroom is usually free of insects, but if you use penny buns, make sure to clean them thoroughly. If you don't live close to a forest, you can make your mushroom outing at the grocery store. The mushrooms sold there are usually free of insects.

Mushrooms with nice caps
Oil
Chopped garlic
Salt
(Filling if you want, like grated cheese and ham)

Marinate the garlic in oil.
    Heat the grill. Wait until it has a nice glow.
    Brush the top of the mushroom caps with the garlic oil. Salt.
    Place the mushroom caps on the grill with the oiled side facing up. This way, we are pre-grilling the underside of the mushroom caps, which ensures a succulent result.
    Turn the mushrooms over after a few minutes and finish grilling them. Top them off with a filling of your choice if you want, or just eat them with olive oil and salt.

One large, grilled cap mushroom contains 2–3 grams of carbohydrates. If you fill them with cheese, olive oil, and ham, the fat-burning quotient will be approximately 1.2.

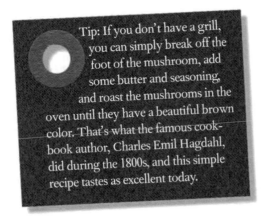
Tip: If you don't have a grill, you can simply break off the foot of the mushroom, add some butter and seasoning, and roast the mushrooms in the oven until they have a beautiful brown color. That's what the famous cookbook author, Charles Emil Hagdahl, did during the 1800s, and this simple recipe tastes as excellent today.

Cauliflower and cheese gratin

Cauliflower is an excellent and useful addition to any healthy meal. You can cook it in lightly salted water and serve it with butter, or you can mix it with butter and cream and make mashed cauliflower. You also have the option to chop it up raw and mix it into a salad. One of the most common ways to prepare this wonderful vegetable is to bake it in the oven with cheese and sauce.

A medium-size cauliflower head
5–7 oz (150–200 g) smoked ham
4 tablespoons crème fraiche
4 tablespoons mayonnaise
About 1¼ cups (300 ml) grated tasty cheese

Preheat the oven to 450°F (250°C).
    Cut the cauliflower into florets and quickly boil them in lightly salted water until they are barely soft. Drain the cauliflower from the water.
    Place the cauliflower florets in a buttered ovenproof dish.
    Mix mayonnaise, crème fraiche, chopped ham, and half of the cheese.
    Spread the mix over the cauliflower and sprinkle the remaining cheese on top.
    Bake in the upper part of the oven until the cheese has a nice color. It takes about fifteen minutes.

3.5 oz (1 hg) of this gratin contains 2 grams of carbohydrates and has a fat-burning quotient of about 1.15. You can eat it on its own or serve it with some sort of meat dish. I like to eat it with sautéed chorizo or lamb sausage. Then you'll get about 6 grams of carbohydrates per serving and a fat-burning quotient of 1.5.

Tip: You can replace the cauliflower with broccoli.

Mashed cauliflower

Boil cauliflower in lightly salted water until it is soft. Drain it from the liquid. Mix the cauliflower with butter and cream until you have a good consistency. If it gets too thin, you can thicken it with cheese and/or egg yolks.
Season with salt and pepper. Add a pinch of nutmeg if you want.

Warm salsa

I've probably made a thousand servings of salsa in the past twenty years. Yes, I even ate salsa during my overweight years. However, it wasn't the salsa that made me obese. I wrote a thorough description about salsa in my previous cookbook, *GI-Zero!* The following is a short version of that.

Habanero peppers, preferably several different varieties.
    Many stores sell a mix of them by the bag.
Yellow onion
Kebab fruits and jalapeno will complement salsa nicely
Sambal oelek is a great spice paste that should be included
Tomatoes and tomato paste simply belong here
In addition, you'll be fine with regular cupboard
    ingredients and a basic spice rack. I'm assuming that
    you normally keep onion, garlic, and lemon at home.
    This salsa is made with a free hand.

I chop the habanero peppers and sauté them in cooking fat. If you don't want the salsa too hot, just take out the seeds. I usually chop up a yellow onion as well. Then I lower the heat and chop up some garlic cloves and add a little bit of crushed tomatoes. Then I'll add a bouillon cube, some tomato paste, and 1 tablespoon of *sambal oelek*. After that I squeeze some fresh lemon juice into the mix! It is absolutely necessary. The secret behind a good salsa is the balance between hot and sour.

I do all this with a free hand. Now it's time to try the salsa. If it is burning like fire on the tongue, I add the remaining crushed tomatoes and perhaps a few coarsely chopped bell peppers. And more lemon. Naturally, more salt and pepper too. Then I let everything cook for a while. At the end, I usually add cumin, ground coriander, and sometimes a tablespoon of paprika. Every once in a while, I tend to add oregano too. Just use what you have. Then I place a lid on top and leave it to sit over the turned off heat. Usually, the salsa turns out perfect. Sometimes, I need to add more salt and lemon.

$\frac{2}{5}$ cup (100 g) of salsa contains 3–4 grams of carbohydrates. If the salsa is really spicy, $\frac{2}{5}$ of a cup will seem like a large portion! Fat-burning quotient: 0.9.

Simple coleslaw

Coleslaw is a fatty cabbage salad that I tend to make in large batches and keep covered in a bowl in the fridge. It is excellent with any meats and lasts a long time.

This is how I make my coleslaw:

I stir crème fraiche with mayo, about equal amounts of each, then I season that with French mustard and lemon juice. Then I add finely chopped cabbage (or cauliflower) and a little bit of onion. Then I season with a lot of lemon pepper.

Coleslaw with sauerkraut

The other day, I went to a lecture for future dietitians. Instead of coming home with a gift bag with a flower in it, I received an exclusive lamb sausage from Taylor and Jones in Stockholm. A lot tastier than a tulip!

The sausage had such a wonderful aroma that I had to heat it in a skillet as soon as I got home. But what was I supposed to eat with it? That's when I found a jar of sauerkraut and created this dish. Coleslaw with sauerkraut.

7 oz (200 g) sauerkraut in white wine

$\frac{1}{5}$–$\frac{2}{5}$ cup (50–100 ml) mayonnaise

1 tablespoon French mustard

A pair of chopped kebab fruits

Black pepper

Mix these ingredients while the sausage is cooking in the skillet. Eat and enjoy.

This "coleslaw" has about 3 grams of carbohydrates per serving. Together with 5.3 oz (150 g) of a high-fat, good-quality sausage, sautéed in butter, you'll get about 800 calories. Count on about 4–7 grams of carbohydrates, depending on what type of sausage you are using. A complete meal has about 85 E percent fat, and the fat-burning quotient is over 2. In other words, perfectly healthy!

Annika's broccoli

One of my friends sautéed fish fillets that she had dipped in egg and sesame seeds. She didn't wash out the skillet before cooking the next meal. She used the same skillet to sauté broccoli florets together with some freshly grated ginger, and a little bit of garlic. The result was surprisingly delicious, she thought, so she sent me the recipe.

Sesame seeds, shelled, a few tablespoons is enough
Broccoli, use the frozen kind, it is usually pre-cooked
Freshly grated ginger
Garlic
Salt and freshly ground black pepper
Lemon juice, if you want
Butter for sautéing

Roast the sesame seeds in a dry skillet. Be careful with the heat so you don't burn the seeds. Add some butter and sauté the broccoli. Season with fresh ginger, according to your own preference, and add some pressed garlic. Season with salt and freshly ground black pepper. I also like to add a few drops of fresh lemon juice.

7 oz (200 g) of this delicious side provides you with 200 calories and about 6 grams of carbohydrates. The fat-burning quotient is 1.

Pesto with leafy greens

Normally, pesto is a mix of flavorful leafy greens, nuts, cheese, and olive oil. It is common to add garlic as well. Store-bought pesto is usually made with basil. Green garlic, arugula, ramsons, or blanched nettles are other good options to use in your pesto.

$\frac{4}{5}$–$1\frac{1}{3}$ cups (25–38 grams) greens
$\frac{2}{5}$ cup (about 55–60 grams) nuts of your choice, pine nuts are a safe bet
$\frac{2}{5}$ cup (42 grams) Parmesan
A few garlic cloves, if you like garlic
Salt and black pepper
Olive oil

Mix the dry ingredients and add olive oil until you are satisfied with the consistency. Season and taste. Most of the time, you'll need to add more salt. Dilute with boiling water if you want the pesto to be thinner. One tablespoon of pesto contains about ½ gram of carbohydrates. The fat-burning quotient exceeds 3.

Tip: Replace the olive oil with butter and you'll have pesto butter.

Oven-roasted vegetables

Root vegetable boxes are delicious, but if you are sensitive to carbohydrates, this is a dish you should be careful with. However, you can make tasty boxes with vegetables that grow above ground. Study my carbohydrate table on page 13 and choose vegetables from the lower half.

Here is a simple suggestion:
Grease a shallow, ovenproof dish with butter and olive oil.
   Cut the vegetables of your choice into wedges, i.e. onion, bell peppers, zucchini, radishes, mushrooms, and garlic.
   Pour melted butter over the vegetables and season with salt and pepper.
   Roast in a hot oven (about 425°F/225°C) until the vegetables have a nice color. It takes about 30 minutes.

You can serve this side dish with any animal products. It contains about 3 to 6 grams of carbohydrates per 3.5 oz (1 hg), depending on what vegetables you are using. The fat-burning quotient is a little bit over 1.

Pantry-clearing tapenade

I made a little pail of tapenade the other day and currently eat it with pretty much anything. For the sake of this cookbook, I jotted down the ingredients. Otherwise, I always make these kinds of medleys with a free hand.

Contents (approximately):
$\frac{2}{5}$ cup (46 grams) sundried tomatoes in oil (add some of the oil into the mix)
$\frac{2}{5}$ cup (46 grams) pickled olives, spicy olives will add more tang, black olives add a nice color
$\frac{2}{5}$ cup (45 grams) flavorful cheese
$\frac{2}{5}$ cup (60 grams) mixed nuts
Olive oil
Pickle juice

I mixed everything into a thick blend and diluted it with some pickle juice. You can also use the juice from pickled olives or capers. Any other seasoning isn't necessary. However, garlic and lemon would have been another option. Or sardines/anchovies. Store these types of spreads in tightly sealed jars in the fridge and they will stay good until you've finished the jar. If you mix in any animal-based foods, it won't hold up as long. Yes, I know this is more like a pesto with tomatoes, but I like the sound of tapenade better.

Tip: I usually add the nuts towards the end, so that there are some small pieces to chew.

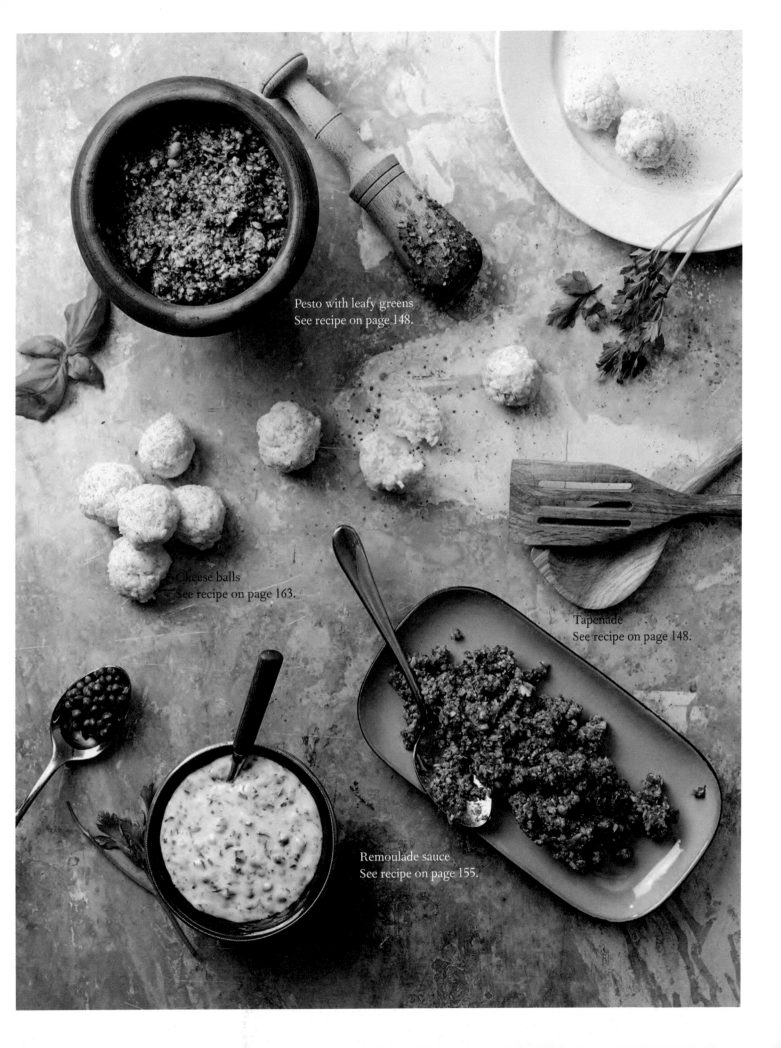

Pesto with leafy greens
See recipe on page 148.

Cheese balls
See recipe on page 163.

Tapenade
See recipe on page 148.

Remoulade sauce
See recipe on page 155.

Tzatziki

The perfect tzatziki is very easy to make. Just soak drained, grated cucumber in garlic yogurt. This recipe is good for four small servings.

1 cucumber
2 garlic cloves (at least)
1¾ cups (about 400 grams) fatty yogurt
5 tablespoons olive oil
2 teaspoons apple cider vinegar
Salt and black pepper

Rinse and cut the cucumber lengthwise. Scrape out the seeds and grate the cucumber coarsely.

Salt the grated cucumber to draw out liquid. You can even leave it in a colander overnight. (Rinse away the salt and press out any excessive water before you use it.)

Peel and press the garlic and mix it into the yogurt with pepper, olive oil, and vinegar.

Add the grated cucumber and season with salt.

One serving of the cooling tzatziki gives about 300 grams calories. The yogurt contains about 5 grams of carbohydrates, the other ingredients are pretty much carbohydrate-free. Unfortunately, you can't make tzatziki without yogurt . . . The fat-burning quotient is 1.6.

How large is a serving?

That depends. If you are growing taller and wider, you'll need more food to grow. Then you'll require a bigger portion than I do. Whoever is eating to lose weight will use up energy from their own body fat. They don't need to eat as much food. The body will get the nutrients it needs anyway.

Olive and feta cheese medley
See photo on page 144.

The Mediterranean kitchen offers many tasty dips that are perfect on a hot summer day, or a great complement to a spicy meal.

3.5 oz (100 g) feta cheese
⅖ cup (45 grams) pimento olives
⅖ cup (25 grams) pitted black olives
1 garlic clove
⅖ cup (about 100 g) fatty yogurt
⅖ cup (about 100 g) crème fraiche
Black pepper

Finely chop the olives. Crumble the feta cheese and mix with olives, pressed garlic, yogurt, and crème fraiche. Season with pepper. The olives and the feta cheese will provide enough salt.

This medley contains about 3–4 grams of carbohydrates per serving, and has a fat-burning quotient that exceeds 2.

Low-carbohydrate zucchini pasta
See photo on page 106.

My favorite recipes change over the years. This past year, "ribbon spaghetti," made from zucchini, has been one of my favorites. I like to eat it with my beloved entrêcote. Sometimes I slice the zucchini directly onto the plate with the meat, but most of the time, I make the pasta separately.

1 large zucchini, or 2 small
1 medium size onion, finely chopped
2 chopped garlic cloves
Butter for sautéing
Salt and pepper

Brown the onion and garlic in butter. Season with salt and pepper.

Use a cheese slicer to peel off the outer layer of the zucchini (with peel on). Don't include the seed layer.

Sauté over medium heat until the zucchini is soft.

3.5 oz (1 hg) of this lovely "pasta" contains about 100 calories and 3 grams of carbohydrates. The fat-burning quotient is about 2.

Tip: Just like any other pasta, you can make a creamed variation by adding cream, crème fraiche, or cheese.

Fried halloumi
Se photo on page 144.

Halloumi is a type of cheese that differs a lot from other cheeses. It originates from Cyprus and used to be made from sheep's milk. Nowadays, it is made in the Mediterranean region with a milk blend from sheep, goat, or cow. The characteristics of the cheese remind me of Sami coffee cheese.

This cheese has a high protein content and you can sauté or grill it the way you cook meat. Use olive oil as cooking fat. Cut the cheese into strips that are about 1.3 inches (½ cm) wide. Heat a skillet with olive oil and fry the cheese until it has a nice color. I like to eat as it is, but some people like to season it with lemon and black pepper. Salt isn't necessary; the cheese is naturally salty.

Halloumi has a fairly low fat content, about 1, but if you sauté it in olive oil, you'll improve the fat value. Count on at least 2 grams of carbohydrates per 3.5 oz (1 hg).

Fake potato salad
See photo on page 153.

Potatoes are excluded as a healthy food option. But, some potato dishes are missed. Potato salad is one of them. My friend, Monica, has provided me with the following recipe, which replaces potatoes with zucchini.

Zucchini, add as much as you need
My mayo sauce, see page 154.
Leek, or red onion
Salt and pepper

Cut the zucchinis in half (peeled or unpeeled), and use a spoon to scoop out the seeds. Cube the zucchini and sauté the pieces in butter until they are soft. Allow to cool.

Make a mayo sauce by combining equal parts mayonnaise and crème fraiche. Season with French mustard and lemon juice.

Finely chop the onion.

Combine everything, season with salt and pepper. I tend to use coarsely ground black pepper. Let the salad sit for a while to allow the flavors to settle.

One serving that is about 7 oz (200 g) contains 5 grams of carbohydrates and has a fat-burning quotient of about 3.

Tip: You can replace the zucchini with radishes.

Cheese gratin with chanterelles

34–68 oz (1–2 liters) freshly plucked chanterelles
10.5–14 oz (300–400 g) flavorful cheese
7 oz (200 g) feta cheese
4 eggs
1¾ cups (400 ml) heavy whipping cream
2 garlic cloves, pressed
2 teaspoons *sambal oelek*
1 yellow onion
Butter for sautéing
Salt and pepper
Parsley

Go chanterelle picking in the forest. Clean the chanterelles.

Chop up the cheese and place it in a greased ovenproof dish.

Make the gratin sauce by beating eggs, heavy whipping cream, garlic, and *sambal oelek*.

Pour the sauce over the cheese and bake in the oven at 400°F (200°C).

Sauté chanterelles with the onion. Season with salt, pepper, and parsley.

Once the gratin has a nice color, remove it from the oven and cover it with the chanterelles before you serve it.

One serving (about 8.8 oz/250 g) contains about 700 calories and 5 grams of carbohydrates. In other words—a complete meal. The fat-burning quotient is about 1.8.

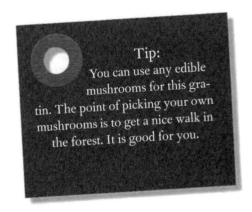

Tip:
You can use any edible mushrooms for this gratin. The point of picking your own mushrooms is to get a nice walk in the forest. It is good for you.

Bread

Crisp bread

Those who have eaten themselves to sickness by excessive consumption of carbohydrates should be careful with bread and foods similar to bread. Even "bread" that contains few carbohydrates contributes to a bread eating habit. Even prefabricated low-carb products contain a lot of carbohydrates.

There are many recipes for low carbohydrate nut and fiber breads. Here is one of them, for a "crisp bread":

¼ cup (40 grams) crushed linseeds
¼ cup (40 grams) hulled sesame seeds
⅘ cup (120 grams) psyllium seed husks
1 teaspoon salt
1 teaspoon bread spices (optional)
2 cups (½ liter) water

Combine the ingredients in a bowl and allow the dry ingredients to absorb the water for a few minutes.

Pour the batter onto a baking tray that has been covered with parchment paper. Flatten the batter evenly.

Bake at 320°F (160°C) until the bread is dry. It takes about an hour.

After about 30 minutes, you can trace squares in the bread, so that it is easier to break into pieces when it is done. You'll get about 16 pieces on a baking tray.

How many carbohydrates does this type of bread contain? And how many of those carbohydrates do we use up? No one knows exactly, but count on at least 1 gram per piece. If you spread enough butter and cheese on top, the small amount of carbohydrates won't raise your blood sugar levels significantly. This type of bread won't make you obese, but it will help you keep your bread-eating habit. That can become an issue when you run out of low-carbohydrate bread options.

The most delicious LCHF bread?

When I lectured at *Finnskogtoppens Helsesenter* (a health center) in Norway, someone presented what I would describe to be the most delicious low-carbohydrate bread I've eaten in my life. Normally I don't eat bread, not even the kinds with few carbohydrates, but a slice of this bread won't make you feel bad. The nutritional value is so great that you could pretty much live off of this bread.

½ tablespoon psyllium husk (can be found in the gluten-free section)
⅖ cup (100 ml) water
⅗ cup (85 grams) crushed linseeds
⅘ cup (about 115 grams) sunflower seeds
1 cup (140 grams) shredded coconut
7 oz (200 grams) finely chopped almonds
4 eggs
2 tablespoons coconut oil (or 3 tablespoons butter)
½ tablespoon Urbase Extra (basic mineral alkaline powder, optional)
½ teaspoon salt

Heat the oven to 320°F (160°C). Mix psyllium husk with water and let it soak in the liquid for five hours. Add linseeds, sunflower seeds, coconut, and almonds. Stir. Then you can add the remaining ingredients. Knead the dough and fill a baking pan or shape into a round boule. Bake for about one hour at the bottom of the oven. This tastes absolutely delicious with butter and flavorful cheese.

One slice of bread that weighs about 1.8 oz (50 g) contains less than 3 grams of carbohydrates. About 80 percent of the energy content (200 calories) comes from fat. This bread contains a great deal of vitamins and minerals, and it has a large fat content. The fat-burning quotient (only the bread) is about 1.8, so it is very healthy. Add some butter and cheese and you'll improve the fat-burning quotient!

P.S. The original recipe also calls for 1 teaspoon cinnamon and ½ tablespoon of cardamom; however, I consider those to be holiday spices.

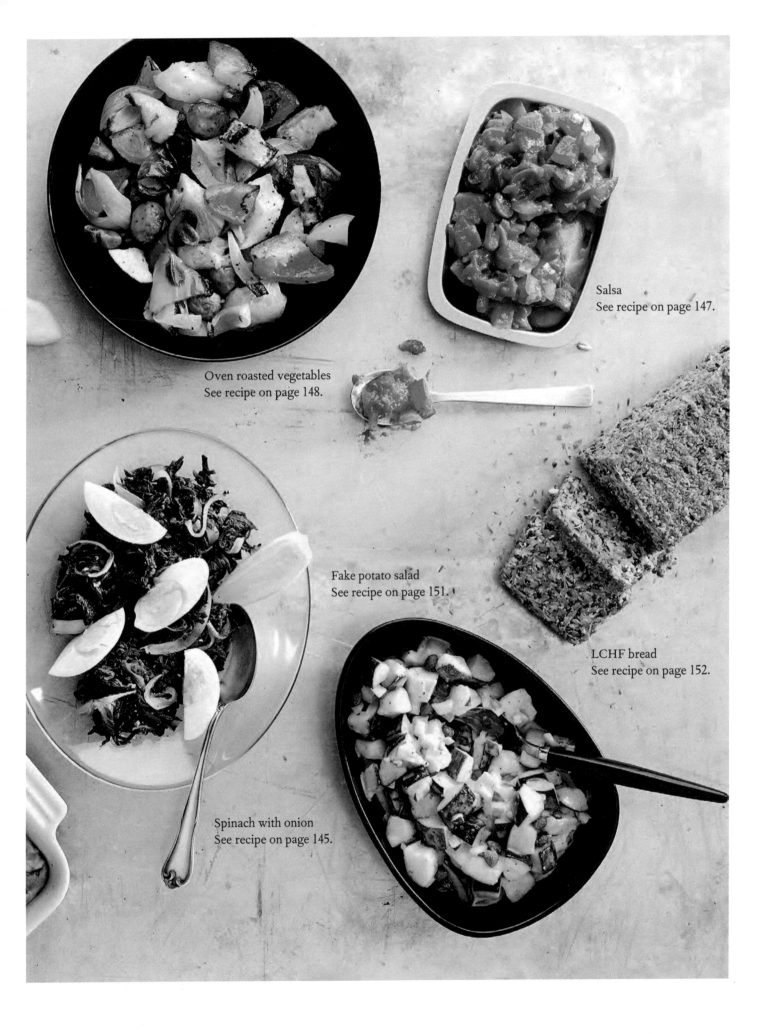

Salsa
See recipe on page 147.

Oven roasted vegetables
See recipe on page 148.

Fake potato salad
See recipe on page 151.

LCHF bread
See recipe on page 152.

Spinach with onion
See recipe on page 145.

Cold sauces and dressings

Sure, butter is great when it melts on a warm steak, or fish. But many other courses are even tastier if you add a creamy sauce, or a delicious butter sauce. Or why not add a cold stirred sauce where fats and acids balance each other out? The nice thing about our new traditional diet is that we don't need to fear fatty sauces.

MAYONNAISE AND MAYO SAUCE: The base for all tasty cold sauces almost always consists of mayonnaise and crème fraiche, in one or another combination. At least according to my taste buds. Sometimes I use only mayonnaise, or only crème fraiche as a starting point, but other times I'll even use sour cream. These type of sauces contain a maximum of 2 grams of carbohydrates per serving, sometimes only half of that. Compare that to store-bought sauces, such as gravlax sauce, that can contain up to five times as many carbohydrates. I love gravlax, but definitely with a sugar-free sauce, such as dill mayo sauce spiked with French mustard and lemon. Sugared sauces don't belong in a healthy diet.

If you want some variation, you can flavor mayonnaise with almost anything; it is very forgiving. The many different seasoning options sometimes give names to new sauces.

Simple mayonnaise

It is very easy to make your own classic mayo. You'll need:

2 egg yolks
2 teaspoons white wine vinegar, or lemon
1 teaspoon French mustard
1⅓ cups (300 ml) cooking oil, don't use flavorful extra
    virgin olive oil!
Salt and pepper

In a bowl, combine all the ingredients except for the oil. Add the oil by the drop in the beginning and whisk thoroughly. When the sauce begins to thicken, pour the oil in a thin stream. Continue adding it until you are satisfied.

Season to taste. If the mayonnaise becomes too thick, dilute with lemon juice or water.

Tip: Press a couple of garlic cloves and you'll have aioli sauce!

Tip: If you buy mayo at the store, make sure it contains 2 grams of carbohydrates per 3.5 oz (100 g) at the most. That's about 0.4 grams of sugar per tablespoon of mayo, and that we can handle.

Sean Connery sauce

An exciting name for an exciting sauce.

1–2 egg yolks
2 tablespoons Japanese soy sauce
½ tablespoon rice vinegar
2 garlic cloves
2–3 tablespoons freshly grated ginger
½ teaspoon sesame oil
1–2 teaspoons *sambal oelek*
1 cup (240 ml) grapeseed oil, or olive oil

Combine ingredients just like in the mayo recipe, adding the oil at the end, at first by the drop, and eventually in a nice thin stream that gradually gets thicker. Keep this sauce in a tightly sealed jar in the fridge.

This sauce/dressing is excellent with almost anything. It makes a tasty dip and adds nice flavor to anything from the grill.

Where does the name come from? One explanation is that the sauce is grayish, plump, and tasty just like Sean Connery?!

I think that's a mean description.

The truth to be told, the sauce is fat (not plump), with a fat-burning quotient that exceeds 10, and with only 1 gram of carbohydrates per serving. A sauce for all attractive, healthy people in other words!

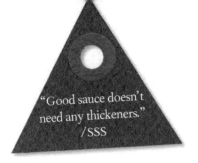

Remoulade sauce

⅘ cup (about 200 ml) mayonnaise
1 tablespoon finely chopped pickle (salty kind)
1 tablespoon chopped capers
1 tablespoon chopped parsley

Combine the mayonnaise with the other ingredients. Eat and enjoy! Capers contain a whole lot of carbohydrates, but you'll still only consume about 2 grams per serving.

Green mayo

⅘ cup (about 200 ml) mayonnaise
1 tablespoon blanched, finely chopped spinach
1 tablespoon chopped leafy herbs, like tarragon or chervil
1 tablespoon chopped parsley

Combine mayo with the remaining ingredients. This sauce is excellent with any cold seafood dishes. It contains less than 1 gram carbohydrates per serving and a fat-burning quotient that exceeds 25!

Versatile cold sauce

When you want a sauce that goes well with anything: Mix crème fraiche with lumpfish roe, finely chopped onion, and lemon. This tastes yummy with anything that has fins, avocado, eggs, and it also makes a very tasty salad dressing. If you want to make it extra luxurious, add some vendace roe.

The cauldron witch's horseradish sauce

Kastrullhäxan (the cauldron witch) is the name of a very nice truck stop restaurant, close to Valla in Sörmland. When I was there, I ate cured salmon with a delicious horseradish sauce that had a lot of tang. I asked the chef for the recipe, like I always do. She responded that she didn't use a recipe, but that she simply combined a lot of freshly grated horseradish with crème fraiche and then added some pepper and a hint of lemon. That's how you make the perfect horseradish sauce!

⅖ cup (100 g) crème fraiche
Freshly grated horseradish (according to your own preference),
   I use about ⅕ cup. That makes it very spicy!)
1 tablespoon freshly squeezed lemon juice
Black pepper
Salt, if you feel like it

This horseradish sauce is excellent with anything from the animal kingdom. One serving contains about 180 calories, a few grams of protein, 17 grams of fat, and 4.4 grams of carbohydrates. Fat-burning quotient: 2.5.

Dressings

What's the difference between a dressing and a sauce? I think the consistency is the biggest difference. If you dilute any kind of flavorful sauce, you'll get a good base for a tasty dressing. Season, and you'll have a mouthwatering dressing.

Jar dressing

When my mayo jar begins to look empty, I stir in a tablespoon of French mustard, add a little bit of vinegar, and some oil. Then I seal with a lid and shake the jar vigorously. If my mustard jar begins to look empty, I do the same thing, but add mayo instead of mustard. You can also add some leafy herb seasoning. That's my simple mayo dressing. It is quick, simple, inexpensive, and the process doesn't even leave any dishes for you to wash! If you want the dressing to be creamier, add some cheese. If you want to dilute it, just add a little bit of water. Count on about 1 gram of carbohydrates per serving. My jar dressings usually have a fat-burning quotient of 10 or more.

Jar vinaigrette is the same thing, except that it doesn't contain any mayo. Use an almost empty mustard jar (sugar-free mustard, of course) and add one part vinegar and four parts oil. Then you shake the jar.

Classic vinaigrette ingredients:

1 teaspoon French mustard
⅖ cup (100 ml) vinegar
1¾ cups (400 ml) oil
Salt and pepper

I usually add a bit more mustard to my dressing and that's usually enough as far as seasoning goes. French mustard is very flavorful on its own.

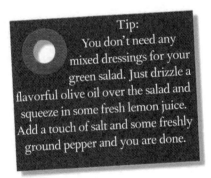

Tip:
You don't need any mixed dressings for your green salad. Just drizzle a flavorful olive oil over the salad and squeeze in some fresh lemon juice. Add a touch of salt and some freshly ground pepper and you are done.

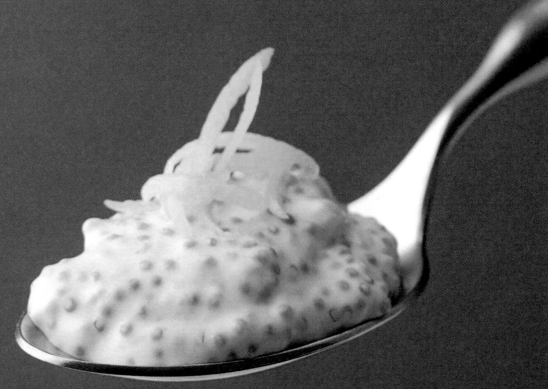

Versatile cold sauce

"All sauces benefit from a dollop of butter at the end."
/SSS

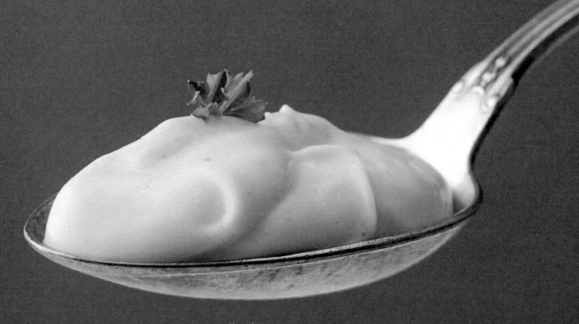

Hollandaise Sauce

Healthy warm sauces

Ten years ago, I ate to achieve health. It was a journey full of pleasure. One of the things that made me really happy about my new diet was all the high-fat, creamy sauces I was allowed to eat. They were tasty and full of flavor. During my obese years, I only ate low-fat sauces, if I allowed myself to enjoy any sauce at all. The very lean cuisine was one of the reasons I couldn't lose any weight. The explanation is simple. Low-fat food contains a lot of carbohydrates, and carbohydrates slow down the fat-burning process.

I make most sauces from scratch. However, I do buy heavy whipping cream, which makes for an excellent sauce on its own with some dishes. I often buy mayonnaise, which is also a type of sauce. On my store-bought list, you can also find Worcestershire sauce (which tastes great in meat pies), Japanese soy sauce, HP sauce, and a few different types of horseradish sauce. Right now you can find Total Insanity and Mama Africa's Zulu Sauce in my pantry. A few drops of spicy horseradish sauce is delicious with eggs and gives the salsa some tang.

WARM BUTTER SAUCES: Béarnaise and hollandaise are warm sauces made with butter. Use the same steps as when making mayonnaise, but heat the sauce and use butter instead of oil. We can refer to this as warm, flavored mayo. In other words, it's all about making an emulsion where little butter bubbles are sustained in liquid. Just like with the mayo, you begin with the egg yolks and something sour, and you beat some fat into this blend.

Heat can create a problem while you cook the sauces. If you allow the sauce to boil, it will separate. That's why it is recommended to cook it in a water bath. If the sauce separates, remove the pot from the heat and add cold liquid. This usually takes care of the problem. If it doesn't, you'll have to start from scratch.

Don't let this scare you away from trying. I make my butter sauces with a free hand, and they never separate. That's because I watch the heat like a hawk. I usually "cook" the sauce on the remaining heat after I turn off the hotplate. A gas stove is on my wish list!

The simplest sauce with sautéed meals

Most of the time I use whatever I'm cooking to flavor my sauces. I put the food on a plate, raise the heat, and pour cream into the skillet. In less than a minute, I have a delicious, flavorful cream sauce. If the sauce needs some more tang, I add Japanese soy sauce, *sambal oelek*, French mustard, or anything else that would go well with the meal. Anchovy juice, capers, and lemon are other options.

If you want the sauce to taste similar to the stroganoff sauce, use onion, tomato paste, crème fraiche, and lemon juice. If you want it to resemble béarnaise sauce, you'll need vinegar, onion, and tarragon. There are endless possibilities. Sometimes I cheat by using store-bought fond.

Hollandaise sauce

Approximately 2.6–3.5 oz (75–100 g) butter
3–4 egg yolks
⅖ cup (100 ml) heavy whipping cream
⅖–⅗ cup (100–150 ml) concentrated fish broth
A splash of white wine, and a few drops of lemon juice
1 tablespoon French mustard, salt, and white pepper
    according to your own preference
2–3 tablespoons parsley, preferably fresh

Melt half of the butter in a small pot. Remove it from the heat. Add egg yolks and cream while you beat the mixture with a whisk. Simmer the sauce in a water bath while you beat it vigorously. As the sauce thickens, add some of the fish broth to achieve a nice consistency. Simmer the sauce. Remove the pan from the heat. Add mustard, lemon, and wine. Then add the remaining butter in lumps while beating the sauce with a whisk. Keep the sauce warm in a water bath (don't cover with a lid).

Tip: Don't allow too much of the liquid to evaporate when you cook the sauce—that will leave nothing for the butter bubbles to float in, and the emulsion separates. Here too, you can solve the issue by adding more liquid. Hollandaise is the mild mother of butter sauces, béarnaise—her famous daughter. The difference is that you use lemon juice, egg yolks, and butter as your base for hollandaise, while the béarnaise is seasoned with vinegar, onion, tarragon, and parsley.

Simple béarnaise sauce

⅘ cup (200 g) crème fraiche
⅖ cup (100 g) mayonnaise
1 finely chopped shallot
1 tablespoon white wine vinegar
1–2 tablespoons dried tarragon
⅖ cup (1 dl) parsley, finely chopped
1 teaspoon Dijon mustard
½ teaspoon salt
Freshly ground white pepper

Combine everything and store the sauce in a cool place. Then cook something to eat with the sauce, perhaps something that used to move.

Traditional béarnaise sauce

I make my béarnaise the traditional way. Follow the recipe a few times and eventually you'll be able to make the sauce with a free hand. I always make sure to have half-melted butter at hand, about 7 oz (200 g), and then I crack some egg yolks into a glass. After that, I'm ready to begin.

I cook a base for the sauce with a few tablespoons of finely chopped onion, some white wine (about ⅖ cup/100 ml), and a few tablespoons of white wine vinegar. Salt and a few crushed white peppercorns. And tarragon, of course! Without tarragon, there is no béarnaise. I often add a little bit of chopped parsley as well. I let the base boil down until only a few tablespoons remain. A proper person would strain this base through a sieve, but I don't.

I set the pan aside and allow it to cool off a bit before I whisk a pair of egg yolks into the pot. Usually this thickens the sauce immediately. Then I place the pan back on the stove and use the heat that lingers once you turn the stove off, and I whisk in some dollops of butter. Do it carefully in the beginning and increase the dollops as you go. Usually the sauce thickens nicely without any issues. Keep in mind that the sauce shouldn't boil; if anything, you may let it half-simmer. If the sauce begins to separate, I add more liquid. You can use vinegar, lemon, white wine, or a little bit of cold water. Or simply an ice cube.

Tip: Once your sauce is cold, you can mix in some butter and you'll have a perfect béarnaise butter with your beef. Also feel free to chop up some parsley and mix it in at the end.

Carrot béarnaise

This is guaranteed to be a different kind of "béarnaise sauce" that most people will like, but that some people can't stand. I have tried it with lamb, chicken, and pork with huge success.

4 carrots (approximately 400 g)
5–8 fresh tarragon sprigs
⅕ cup (50 ml) white wine vinegar
3.5 oz (100 g) butter, room temperature
Shallot and pepper

Slice the peeled carrots and boil them until soft in lightly salted water. Drain.

Remove the leaves from the tarragon sprigs and set them aside.

Boil the sprigs in the vinegar, until half of the liquid has evaporated. Remove the sprigs.

Combine the drained carrots with the vinegar, tarragon leaves, and butter.

Season with salt, pepper, and optionally, more tarragon. Heat the sauce right before you serve it.

This sauce isn't as low in carbohydrates and doesn't contain as much fat as the other sauces, but you still won't consume more than 4 grams of carbohydrates per serving. The fat-burning quotient is about 2.

Simple green pepper sauce

In a saucepan, sauté a couple of tablespoons of green pepper with finely chopped onion. I recommend using butter as cooking fat. Once the onion turns transparent, add about 1¾–2 cups (400–500 ml) heavy whipping cream, lower the heat, and boil the sauce until only half of it remains. Season and flavor with Japanese soy sauce, fond, or cognac. Or just use the cooking fat from whatever you just cooked.

Tip: The easiest way to make pepper sauce is by rubbing your meat (or whatever you may be cooking) with pepper (be generous) before you sauté it. When the food is almost cooked, add cream to the skillet and you'll have a delicious sauce.

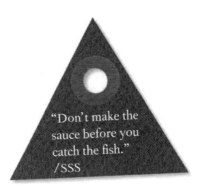

"Don't make the sauce before you catch the fish."
/SSS

Two shrimp sauces

I make two types of shrimp sauce, one cold and one warm. The cold sauce I make with shrimp, crème fraiche, cream, fish roe, and lemon. Improvised proportions. When I'm feeling more elegant, I use lightly beaten cream. Otherwise, I just add cream to dilute the sauce until it has a desirable consistency. If I want some heat, I add a little bit of *sambal oelek* (a chili paste). Count on about 2 grams of carbohydrates per serving.

The warm shrimp sauce is a classic, and I've mentioned it in many of my previous cookbooks. However, it is so delicious that I'm going to share the recipe with you again. Just like any authentic shrimp sauce, this one is based on a fond (don't use the store-bought kind). Fond is a type of broth that has boiled down. No store-bought fond will ever come close to the homemade kind. Luckily, the shrimp fond is really easy to make.

Making a broth or fond can take forever when you cook it off of meat and bones. The shrimp fond only takes about 30 minutes. It is quick and inexpensive, because you use shrimp heads, roe, and peel to make the base. If you keep a jar of shrimp fond in the fridge or freezer, you can always impress your guests as a master chef and quickly throw together a mouthwatering shrimp sauce or shrimp soup. Save the shrimp to decorate your pike mousse, or to throw into your shrimp soup. If you are making the fond for future use, you can eat the shrimp with something nice, such as mayonnaise, egg, and asparagus. A little lovely lunch like that contains 3–4 grams of carbohydrates, depending on how much lemon you use. The fat-burning quotient is about 2.5.

For the fond:
2.2 lbs (1 kg) shrimp with peel
Cooking fat (butter or oil)
2 yellow onions
2 tablespoons tomato purée
34 oz (1 liter) fish broth
4/5–2/5 cup (100–200 ml) dry white wine (optional, but delicious)
Spices of your choice, such as parsley, chervil, paprika, tarragon

For the sauce/soup:

Heavy whipping cream, according to need. I use about 17 oz (0.5 liter).

Making the fond: Peel the shrimp and put it aside. Fry the shrimp meat and roe in butter or olive oil. Don't mind the smell! Add finely chopped onion and the other ingredients once the peel begins to pale. Dilute with broth and wine. Now the basic work is done. Traditional cooking is simple!

Allow to simmer for 20 minutes before you strain the fond to remove the peel. Now you have a shrimp broth that is the beginning of a fabulous fond. You can freeze the broth as it is for future use, or you can boil it down to shrimp soup/shrimp sauce. To me, they are the same, except that I may add more spices to the sauce than I would to the soup.

Making the soup or sauce: Boil down the shrimp broth until about half of the liquid remains. Dilute the broth with heavy whipping cream, 4/5 cup (200 ml) or more, and simmer the sauce for 15 minutes. Add more cream to achieve a nice consistency. Season with salt, pepper, cayenne pepper, and perhaps a drop of lemon. When I want to eat the sauce as a soup, I add the shrimp that I set aside right before I serve the meal. They should only heat up. Garnish with parsley. If I want to eat it as a sauce, I serve it with Elisabeth's pike and salmon mousse (see recipe on page 79).

If you want a thicker sauce, you can thicken it with egg yolks that have been lightly beaten with heavy whipping cream, not flour. Beat vigorously, and carefully simmer the sauce; don't allow it to boil heavily. You may need to add a lot of egg yolks before you are satisfied with the consistency. However, with each egg yolk, the sauce is even healthier!

Count on 1–2 grams of carbohydrates per 2/5 cup (100 ml) of sauce/soup. The fat-burning quotient for the sauce is about 5; for the soup, about 1. The soup has a lower fat-burning quotient because of the added shrimp, and is very lean and protein-packed. Even protein lowers the fat-burning quotient!

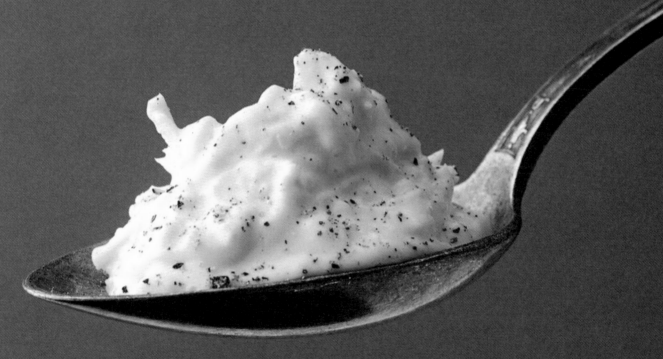

"England has three sauces and three hundred different religions, while France has three religions and three hundred sauces."

/ French proverb

Horseradish cream without cream
See recipe on page 163.

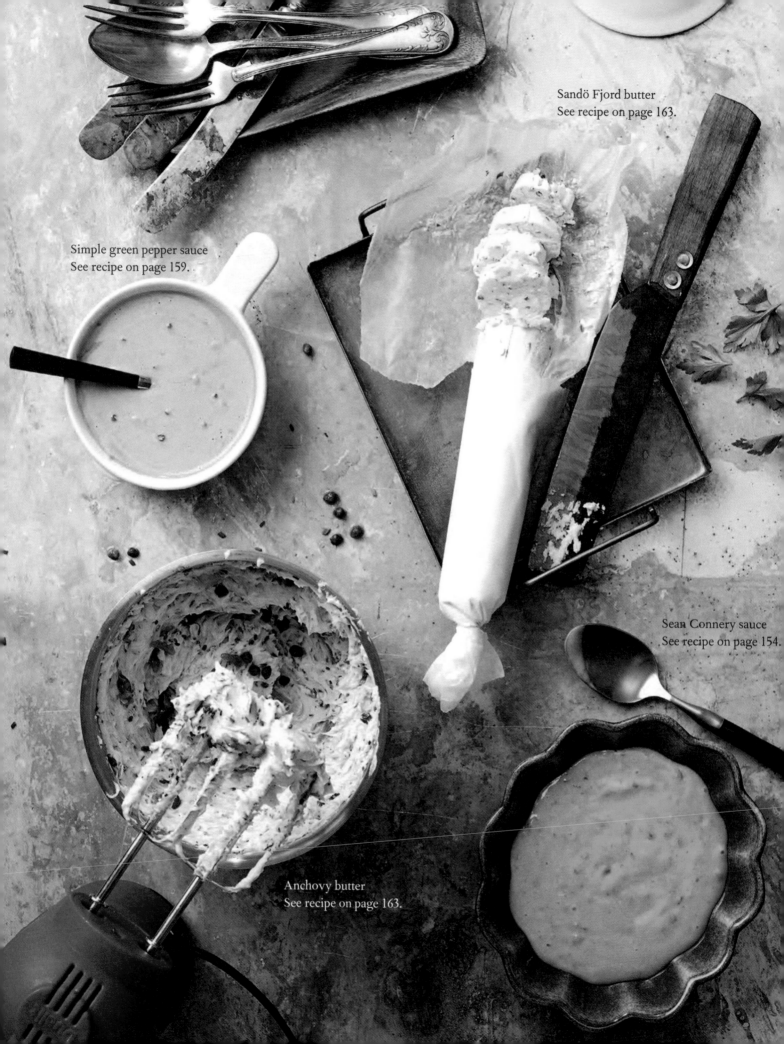

Sandö Fjord butter
See recipe on page 163.

Simple green pepper sauce
See recipe on page 159.

Sean Connery sauce
See recipe on page 154.

Anchovy butter
See recipe on page 163.

Seasoned butter and dips

Aromatic butter

Butter is delicious and healthy, whether you cook with it or garnish your food with it. An aromatic butter can improve the flavor of any animal-based meal. I always keep my butter out at room temperature, which makes it easy to mix with spices. If I'm in a hurry, I may use a cheese slicer to slice cold butter directly over the food, then press a fresh garlic clove on top, and finish off by sprinkling some fling salt (preferably flavored) over everything,

The simplest butter

I combine room temperature butter, salt, (garlic), and chopped parsley. The butter is ready! This is simple parsley butter. If I use dill instead of parsley, I'll have dill butter. The same way, I can exchange the dill for freshly grated horseradish, or replace the horseradish with freshly grated ginger. A few drops of lemon and Worcestershire sauce brings out the flavors even more.

Variation: If I want my butter a bit whiter and fluffier, I'll mix in some cream. Use one part cream for every two parts of butter.

Red wine butter

Red wine butter is flavored with red wine that has been boiled down with onion. Then you'll just season it with spices of your choice. I use salt, pepper, and lemon. Begin by frying finely chopped red onion in butter. You can use a shallot as well, but it won't give the same nice color as the red onion. Add half a bottle of red wine to the onion, and boil down at low heat until most of the liquid has evaporated. Allow the concoction to cool and mix it with butter, or whip it up with a fork. Oftentimes, I also add a handful of finely chopped parsley at the end.

Simple béarnaise butter

The béarnaise sauce has a nice seasoning blend that gets its character from tarragon, parsley, vinegar, crushed white pepper, and shallot. Use the same seasoning to give the characteristics of béarnaise sauce to any mixed dips, such as butter. Combine and salt according to your own preference. Allow the flavors to settle. If you are really thorough, boil the spices down with a little extra water and a few tablespoons of vinegar. Allow the excess liquid to boil down and combine. Then the flavors will settle right away.

Advanced béarnaise butter

Cook a béarnaise sauce according to the instructions in the recipe on page 159. Allow the sauce to cool and mix with the same amount of butter. I usually add lemon and salt at the end as well.

Anchovy butter

Combine butter with anchovies. Use about 1–2 anchovy fillets per $\frac{2}{5}$ cup (100 ml) of butter, and dilute with a little bit of the anchovy liquid. Or, you can simply chop down the anchovy fillets into the butter and stir. Capers and chives complement this butter as well. Season with pepper and lemon juice. The fat-burning quotient is about 15.

Sandö Fjord butter

This classic Norwegian fish sauce is based on heavy whipping cream and butter. It is supposed to be mild. Over low heat, boil down heavy whipping cream until about half of the volume remains in the pan. Turn off the heat and add butter, twice as much as the whipping cream. Once the butter has melted, use a whisk to beat the creamy blend into a fluffy butter. I like to finish off by adding a lot of parsley and a few drops of lemon. Sandö Fjord butter tastes delicious with any type of white fish. If you find this butter to be too bland, spice it up with *sambal oelek*, even though it breaks the rules for this butter.

Cheese balls

No matter what soup I make, I always place some cheese balls in the bowl, or I'll place a bowl filled with an assortment of cheeses in the center of the table. I coarsely grate a flavorful cheese, at least $\frac{1}{5}$ cup (40 g), and then I stir the cheese into a bowl with crème fraiche. It is quite fascinating how much cheese I can fit into that bowl. I'm not satisfied until the batter is so firm that the spoon begins to bend. I only season this medley with cayenne pepper.

Horseradish cream without cream

Grate cheese. Mix it into mayo and crème fraiche. I use more mayo. Then I season with freshly grated horseradish according to my own preference and finish off with some freshly ground black pepper. If I'm serving this cream with roast beef, I'll add a lot of pepper! This "cream" is packed with tang and also tastes great with fish, in which case I also add lemon.

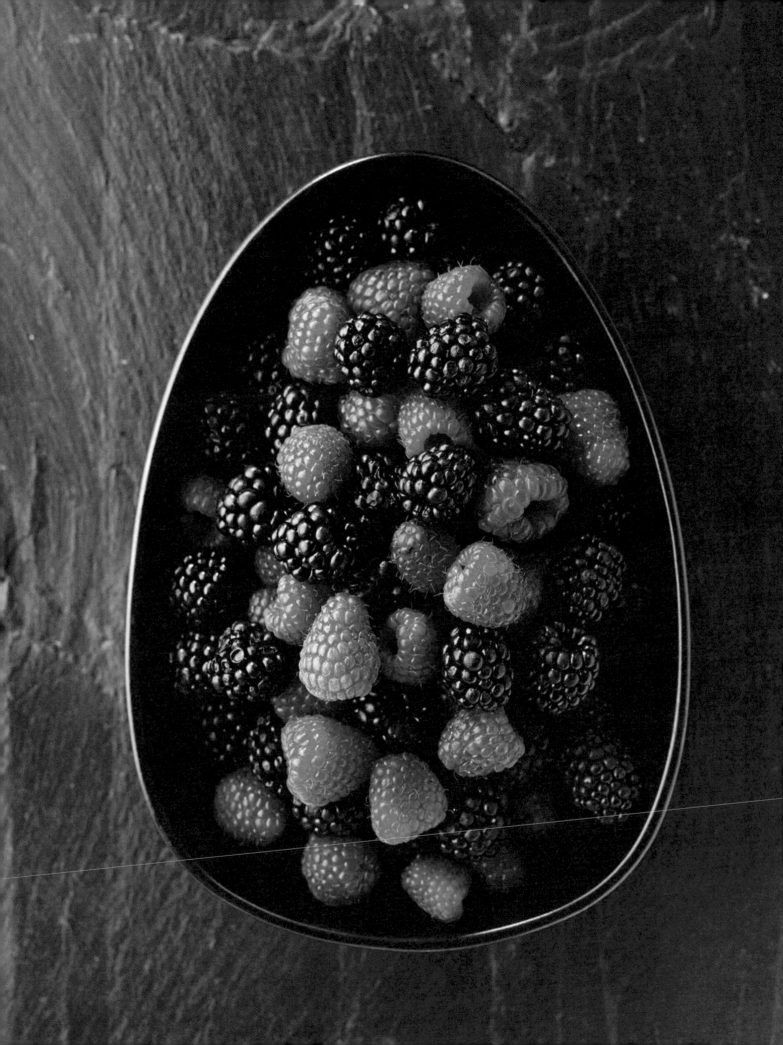

Desserts

High-fat, sugar-free desserts
are almost healthy

7.

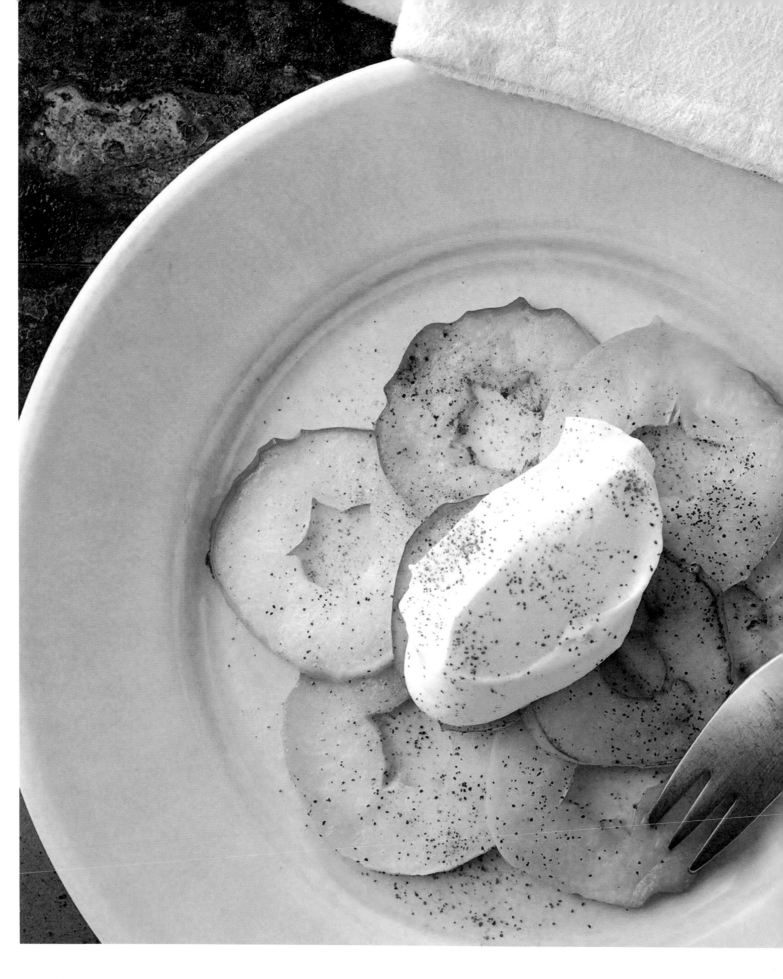

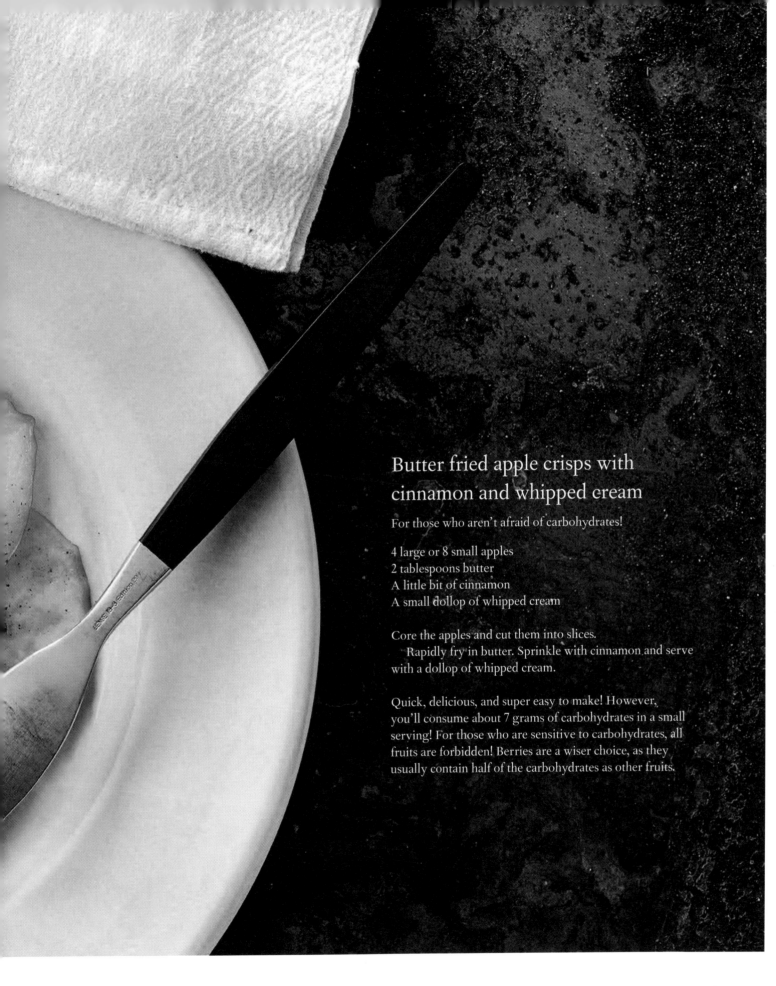

Butter fried apple crisps with cinnamon and whipped cream

For those who aren't afraid of carbohydrates!

4 large or 8 small apples
2 tablespoons butter
A little bit of cinnamon
A small dollop of whipped cream

Core the apples and cut them into slices.
    Rapidly fry in butter. Sprinkle with cinnamon and serve with a dollop of whipped cream.

Quick, delicious, and super easy to make! However, you'll consume about 7 grams of carbohydrates in a small serving! For those who are sensitive to carbohydrates, all fruits are forbidden! Berries are a wiser choice, as they usually contain half of the carbohydrates as other fruits.

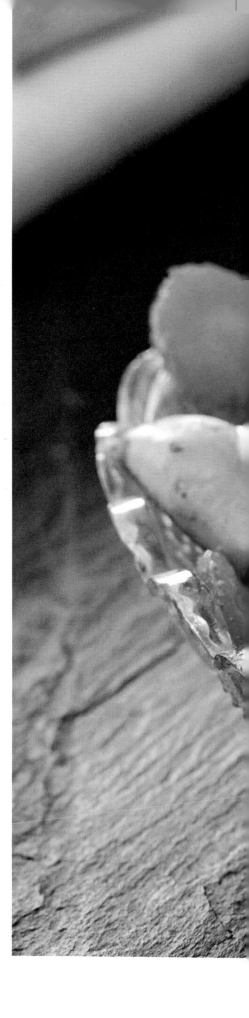

Roasted Brazil nuts with lime-marinated strawberries

For the nuts:
24 Brazil nuts, organic are best
1 tablespoon butter

For the strawberries:
⅖ cup (100 ml) whipped cream
4 beautiful strawberries, preferably with the stems

For the garnish:
½ cup (100 ml) whipped cream
4 nice strawberries with the stems and leaves

Slice the strawberries and combine with lime juice and lime zest. Marinate for 20–30 minutes.
    Roast the nuts in butter, allow to cool.
    Beat the cream.
    On a plate, arrange strawberries and nuts elegantly.
    Pipe some cream on top or add it by the dollops.
Garnish with a whole strawberry if you want.

One serving contains about 340 calories and 7 grams of carbohydrates. It's up to you to decide if you can afford this dessert in your diet.

"Strength is the ability to break a chocolate bar into four pieces with your bare hands—and then eat just one of those pieces."

/ Judith Viorst

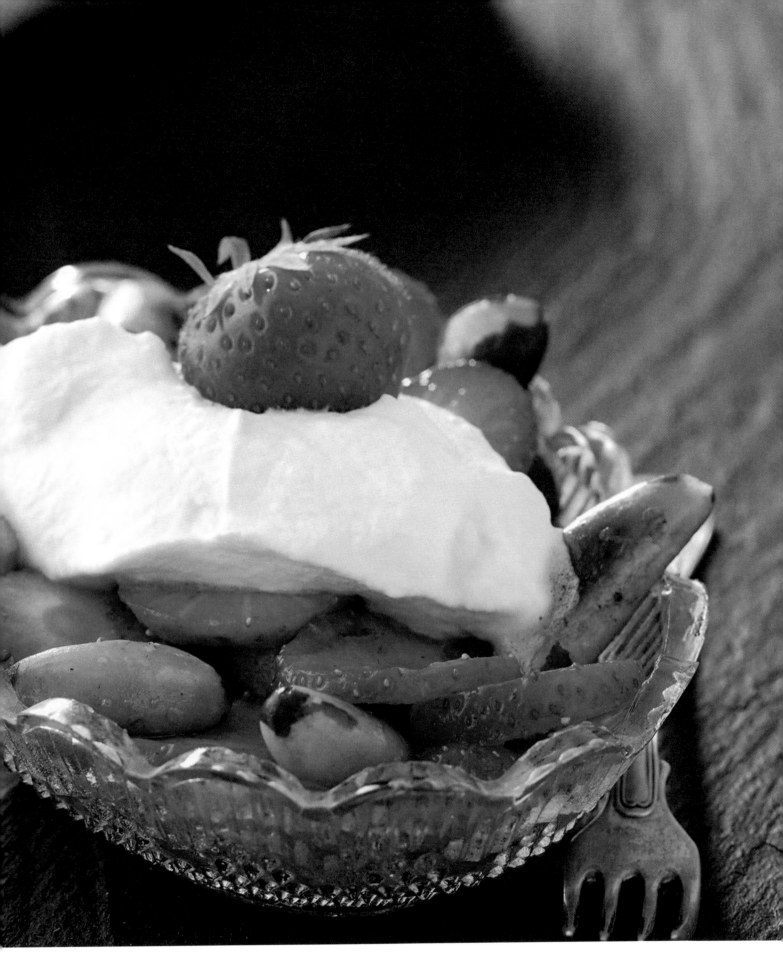

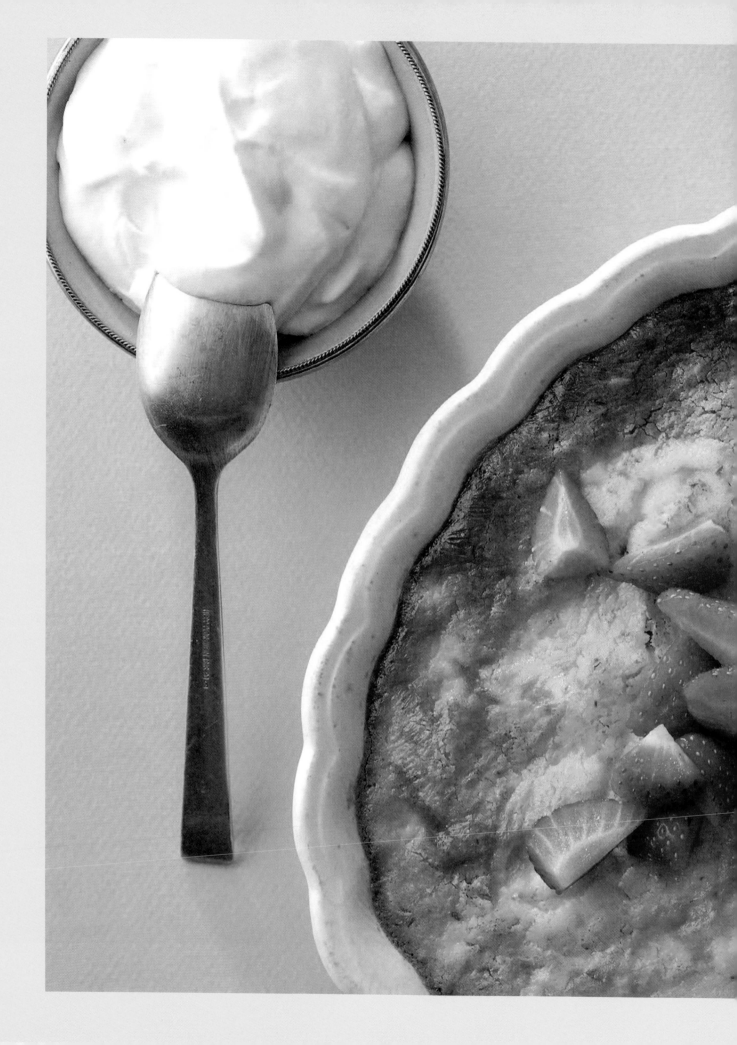

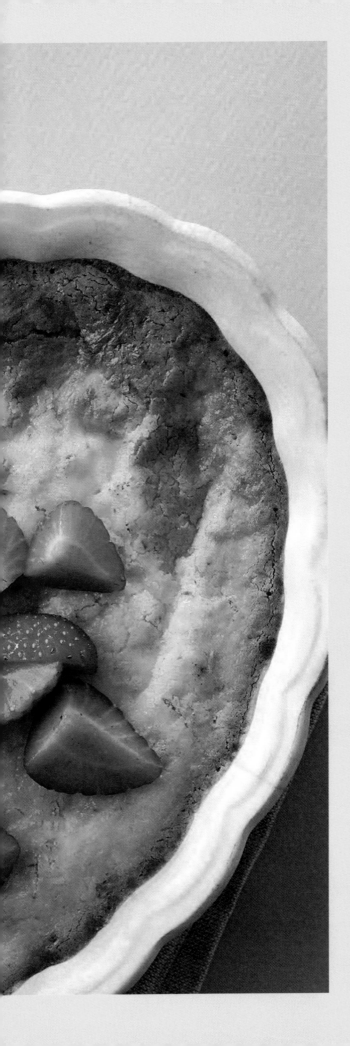

Cheesecake

18 oz (500 g) cottage cheese
³/₅ cup (150 ml) heavy whipping cream
3 eggs
²/₅ cup (45 grams) chopped almonds
Butter to grease the pan
Seasoning of your choice, you can use 1 drop of bitter
    almond oil, the seeds from ½ vanilla pod, lemon zest, or
    ½ gram of saffron.

Drain the cottage cheese for a few hours with a straining-
cloth. If you don't have time for this, use the cheese as it is.
    Combine the ingredients and pour the batter into a
fairly small (7 x 10 in/18 x 25 cm) greased pan.
    Bake at 320–340°F (160–170°C) for approximately
40–45 minutes.

Allow cake to cool for a bit and serve it lukewarm with
fresh or thawed frozen berries and whipped cream.
3.5 oz (100 g) of cheesecake only contains 2.5 grams of
carbohydrates, but you probably won't eat more than
3.5 oz (100 g). Strawberries and whipped cream add some
more carbohydrates, but also some healthy fats. Count
on a big dollop of whipped cream and ¹/₅ cup (30 grams)
berries, and add about 3 grams of carbohydrates.

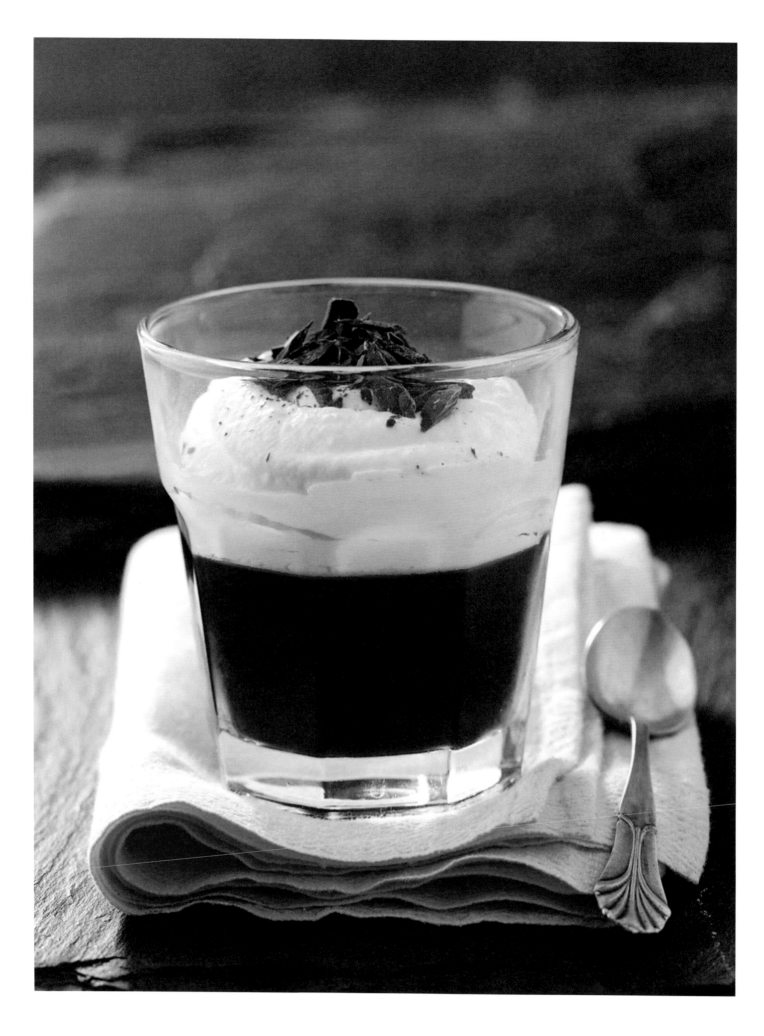

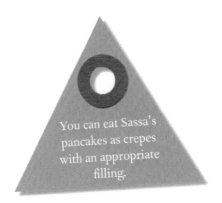

You can eat Sassa's pancakes as crepes with an appropriate filling.

Karen's coffee dessert

1¾ cups (400 ml) delicious, strong coffee
4 teaspoons gelatin powder
⅘ cup (200 ml) heavy whipping cream
1.4 oz (40 g) high-percentage dark chocolate

Make the coffee, stir in the gelatin powder, and transfer to four glasses.

Store in the fridge until it solidifies.

Grate or coarsely chop the chocolate, and beat the cream.

Pipe or dollop the cream on top of the solidified coffee, sprinkle with grated chocolate.

Add as much chocolate as your conscience allows. I suggest about 0.35 oz (10 g) per person. Many people can eat more than that, while others should eat only half of that. ⅖ cup (100 ml) coffee, ⅕ cup (50 ml) whipped cream, and 0.35 oz (10 g) dark chocolate (70%) contains 250 calories and 4.8 grams of carbohydrates. Most of the carbohydrates come from the chocolate.

How large is a serving?

That depends on who you are. I know people that are born with a metabolism that works like fire. They can eat twice as much as I do and remain stick-thin. To them, no portions are too large. If you have eaten yourself to obesity, you need to listen to your body. When you no longer feel hungry, you stop. That's when you know that you have eaten a serving that is just right.

Sassa's pancakes

See photo on page 174.

⅘ cup (200 ml) heavy whipping cream
2 eggs
⅖ cup (100 ml) water
1 tablespoon psyllium husk, allow it to swell in the batter
2 tablespoons melted butter
Salt

Combine everything and cook as thick pancakes. Or make a bacon pancake by pouring the batter into a pan with fried bacon, and bake it in the oven at 350°F (175°C) for 30 minutes. These pancakes turn out so deliciously crispy when you make them thin that they can be eaten on their own or as crepes—with appropriate filling. Shrimp, crème fraiche, and dill are a nice and cooling combination. Ground meat with taco seasoning, grated cheese, onion, and some spicy tomato medley is excellent for anyone that is craving some heat on their tongue. There are endless possibilities.

One batter makes four large, thin pancakes. Each pancake provides less than 2 grams of carbohydrates and has a fat-burning quotient of about 4.5. If you eat it with a few tablespoons of crème fraiche and ⅖ cup (about 60 g) shrimp, you'll have a complete meal with 450 calories, less than 4 grams of carbohydrates, and a fat-burning quotient that is about 2.5. The fat-burning quotient decreases when you fill your crepe because shrimp is full of lean protein. You'll get the fat-burning quotient if you divide the fat weight by the combined gram weight of protein and carbohydrates. Always aim for as few carbohydrates as possible.

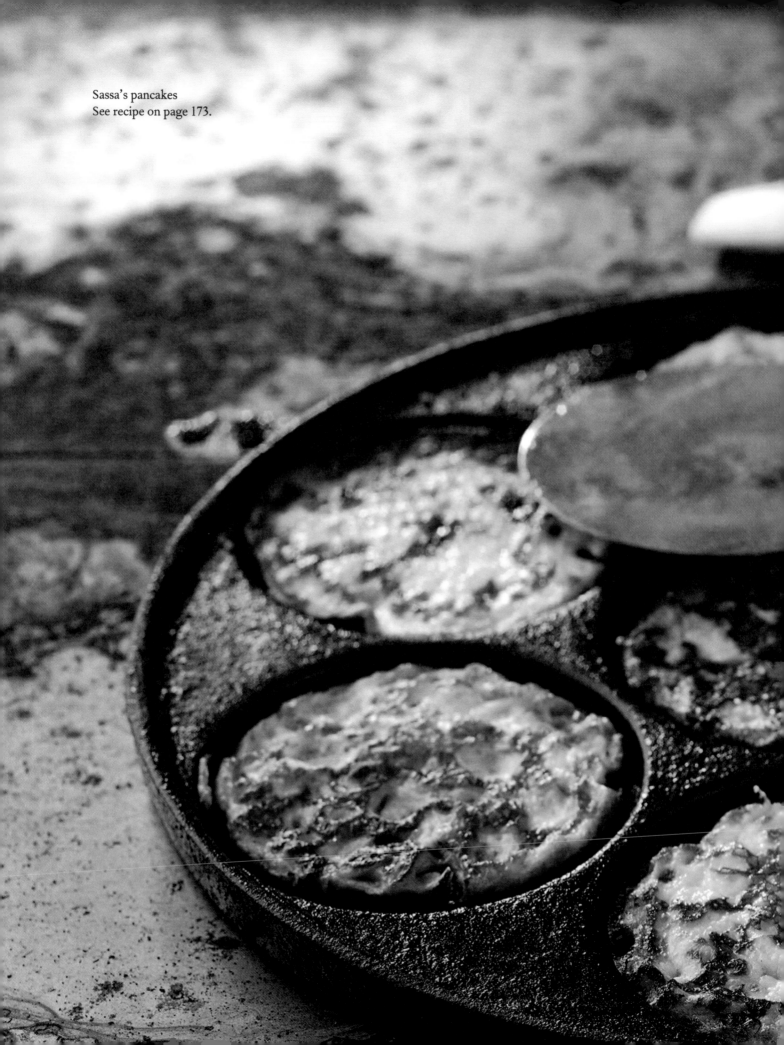

Sassa's pancakes
See recipe on page 173.

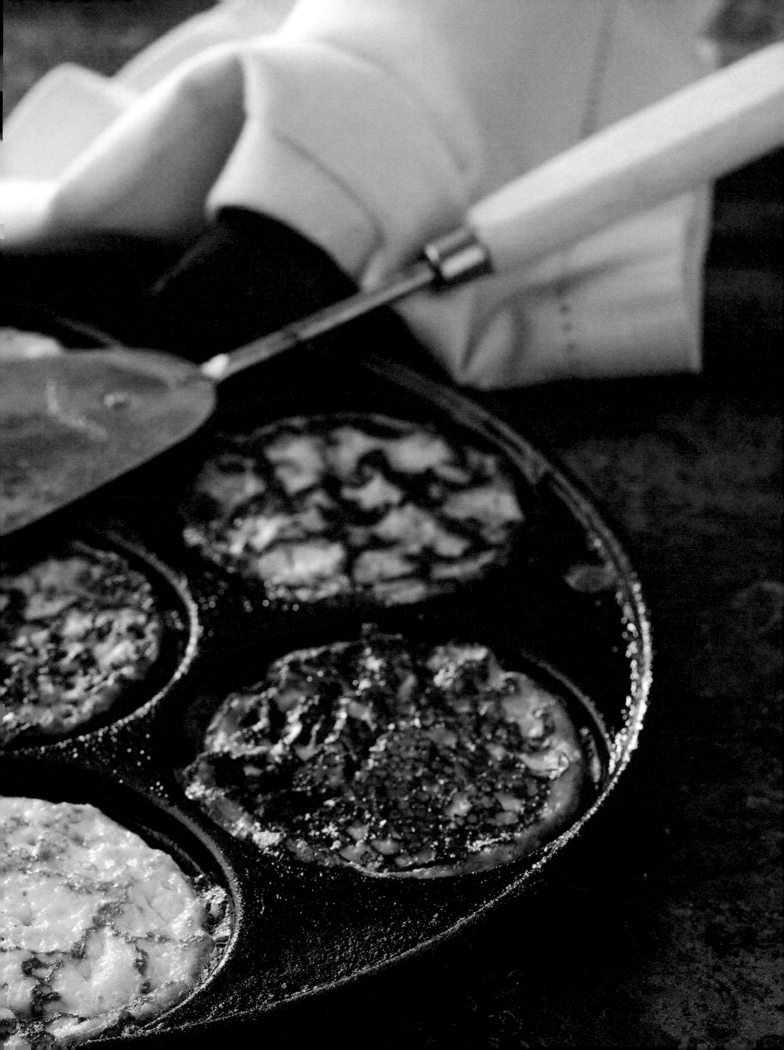

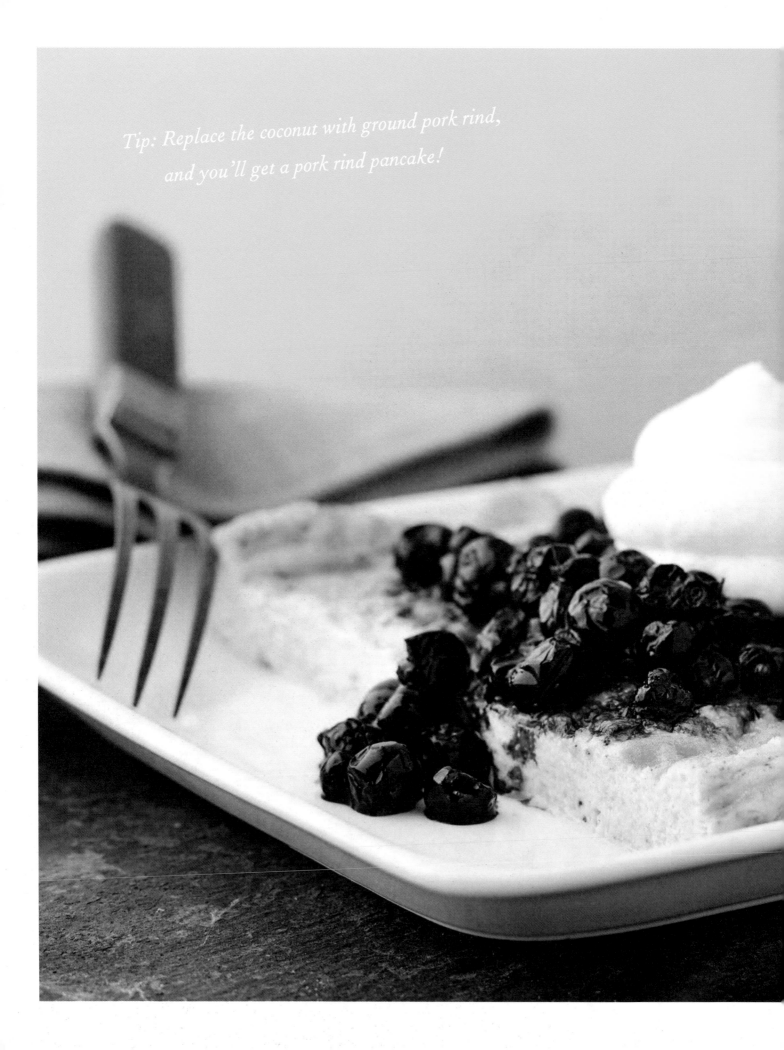

*Tip: Replace the coconut with ground pork rind,
and you'll get a pork rind pancake!*

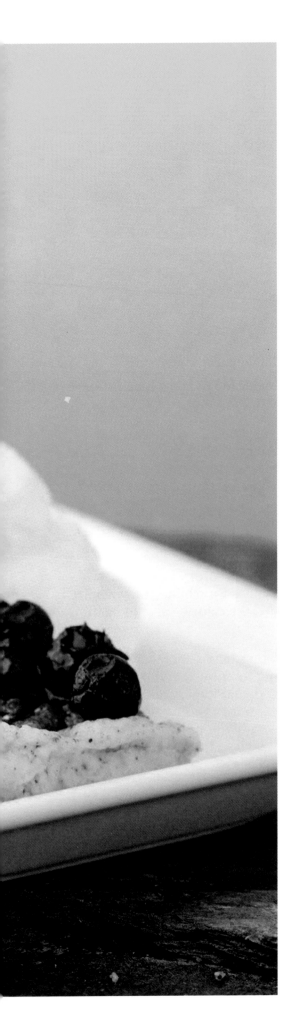

Åland pancake with few carbs

It is difficult to find healthy baked goods that won't spike a sugar rush or insulin. However, this time we've found one. If you like saffron pancakes from Gotland, you'll probably enjoy this variation from Åland as well. I found this recipe online and am grateful to the unknown creator of it.

6 eggs

1⅓ cups (300 ml) heavy whipping cream

1⅓ cups (180 grams) coconut flour, make by running coconut flakes (with few carbohydrates) in a food processor.

½ teaspoon cinnamon

½ teaspoon cardamom (optional)

A pinch of salt

Sweeten with a little bit of stevia if you desire.

Combine all the ingredients and allow time for the batter to swell and for the flavors to settle. Place parchment paper in a medium-sized pan, pour the batter into the pan, and bake in the oven at 400–450°F (200–225°C) until the pancake has a nice color. It takes about 20 minutes.

Traditionally, this Åland pancake is often served cold with whipped cream and jam, but we are skipping the jam. A few frozen raspberries or blueberries as garnish will do.

This pancake is a very nice dessert, or a delicious treat with coffee. It also fits perfectly in the summer picnic basket. If you cut the pancake into nine pieces, you'll get about 2 grams of carbohydrates and a whole daily recommended value of saturated fat per slice. A dollop of cream and a few raspberries add about 1 gram of carbohydrates.

The fat-burning quotient without the cream is 2.5.

A short summary

LCHF/GI-Zero is a natural diet that facilitates stabilized blood sugar levels and a long list of health benefits, such as weight loss. However, the other rewards are even more important.

This is a book about the natural Scandinavian diet that has had huge success in Sweden and Norway for the past few years. Currently it is also taking off in the English-speaking part of the world. With this diet, we have developed a concept that the rest of the world can't quite pigeonhole. I've met many Americans with guru status, and all of them agree that we know best.

The usual term for this diet is LCHF (Low Carb, High Fat), but I often refer to it as GI-Zero! Most important to me is not what the diet consists of, but how it affects our health. In this case, it stabilizes our blood sugar levels. A low GI is good, but GI-Zero is great!

All of the recipes in this book have their nutritional value established according to my knowledge. They give you the carbohydrate and fat-burning quotient values for a bunch of delicious and healthy meals. Just cook and eat. As a bonus, I've also included the calorie value in many of the recipes, but that is far less important to know.

I have to brag a little bit when I say that this cookbook is written by a man with the answer sheet in his hand. I know how to eat to achieve health. It's amazing to know that thousands of other people have found their way to health through my method, and it makes me happy to read their success stories on their journey to good health. If you want to come along on a similar journey, use the recipes in this book to guide you. However, if you just want to eat delicious, healthy, and easy-to-cook meals, this book is for you as well!

A common question: Why does the Swedish government recommend low-fat, industrialized foods that are packed with carbohydrates? Why do they suggest foods that contain artificial fats? Perhaps Larry Hagman was right. The American actor received the same question when he spoke about his health journey on American television the other year. Larry Hagman responded: "They are lying to us!"

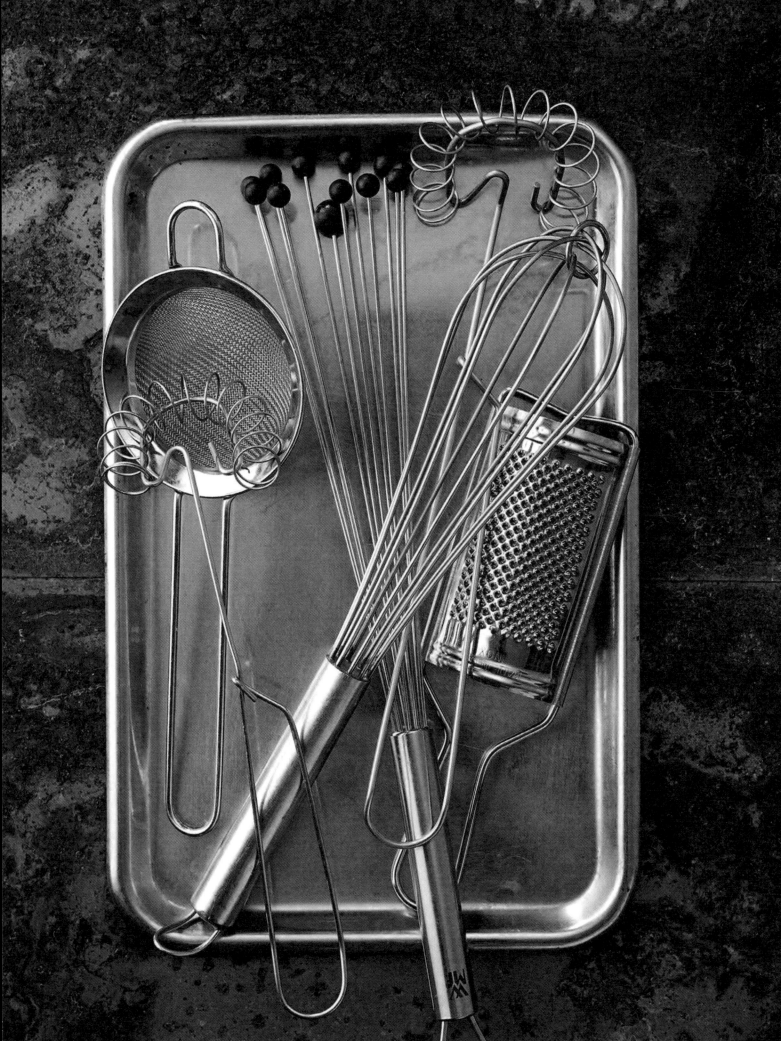

About this book

THIS IS A BOOK about how to eat your way to health by means of delicious and filling food. This is my recipe to health and I've tried it out for many years. Today, hundreds of thousands of other Swedes eat this way too. I know from my own experience that you'll achieve faster and better health results on the LCHF diet than on any other diet that you've tried.

MOST OF IT IS NEW: Most of the recipes in this book are new, but I've also included a few classics from my previous books. An LCHF book without coleslaw or mashed cauliflower is no LCHF book. I've tested most of the recipes out in my own kitchen, but about a third of them come from my dear pen pals and from chefs I know.

ONLY SIMPLE RECIPES: No advanced cooking skills required to cook healthy meals in this book. I've made sure to write simple and straightforward recipes that can be made with basic kitchen tools, with the basic ingredients that most of us have at home. I'll probably write an advanced cookbook in the future, but it won't be this time.

THE HEALTH IS THE IMPORTANT FACTOR: Most of my recipes are based on an animal-based food diet—in other words, things that moved around. The reason behind that is simple. I write about health, and meat contains more nutrients than any vegetable. Simply put, my food philosophy is my health philosophy.

READ MY OTHER BOOKS: If you want to know more about why you should follow this type of diet, you can read my other books to get the whole picture. My most important book is *GI-Noll!* (*GI-Zero!*). The funniest one is probably *Ät dig ner I vikt* (*Lose Weight by Eating*). That's where I tell the amazing tale about a complete amateur who made huge achievements in the world of medicine, but was completely ignored by authorities.

Word references

FAT is one of our most important nutrients, and certainly our most important source of energy. Without fat in our diet, we'll die. Saturated fat is mostly found in animal-source foods, so they are a wise choice. Coconut fat is the best choice in the vegetable kingdom. Monounsaturated fats (olive oil) are another healthy option. Polyunsaturated fats in their artificial form, like margarine and cheap cooking oils, should be avoided.

FAT FUELED: The goal of my diet is to stop our bodies from running on sugar (and easily digested carbohydrates), and start using fat as an energy source. When we use fat as fuel, it is easier to manage a healthy body weight. As a bonus, we get rid of a long list of sugar-related illnesses.

FAT-BURNING QUOTIENT is my own measurement. "Skaldeman's fat-burning quotient" is the value you get when you divide the fat value by the proteins and carbohydrate value in any food. The idea is that the fat should weigh at least as much as the protein, and that the carbohydrate value should be small. Example: If you eat 100 grams of fat, 80 grams of protein, and 20 grams of carbohydrates, you'll get the fat-burning quotient value by dividing 100 by 80 + 20, which is 100. 100 divided by 100 gives us a fat-burning quotient of 1. The higher the fat-burning quotient, the better. To make your life easier, I have provided you with the fat-burning quotient for most of the recipes in the book.

KILOCALORIES (kcal), or calories (as they are referred to), measure how much heat is needed when something is heated in an oven, such as firewood, or pork. There are dieticians that believe our bellies are like ovens. If that were true, we would get fat from eating firewood! The amount of calories that we consume is irrelevant. What matters is what we do with those calories, and how satisfied we feel. I've included the calorie count in the recipes where the serving sizes are established.

CARBOHYDRATES are nutrition-less turbo fuel. They are great for people who run marathons, or dig ditches by hand. People like that need a lot of energy. The problem with carbohydrates is that they slow down the fat-burning process in our body. People who don't lead an active lifestyle and consume a lot of carbohydrates turn off their natural fat-burning process and therefore become obese and undernourished at the same time.

PROTEINS are our building blocks. Your greatest source of protein comes from animal-source foods. Without proteins, your physique collapses. But don't feed your body more proteins than it needs, especially if you are overweight. Then it is better to use fat for energy fuel, both the fat that you consume by mouth, and the fat reserves in your body.

Sugar leads to diabetes

We've increased our sugar consumption by one hundred times in a century! Our intake of refined sugars has increased from 2.2 lbs (1 kg) to 99 lbs (45 kg). Not to mention the same amount of sugars that are hidden in different industrially produced foods under a hundred different names. When I was a child, we used to drink approximately 338 oz (10 liters) of soda each year. Our parents consumed less than that. Diabetes used to be rare back then. Today, we consume several thousand ounces of soda per person each year, and diabetes has become an epidemic.

Add the amount of easily digested starches that exist in prefabricated foods, and you'll get even more sugar. Starch is converted to sugar in the mouth. Industrially produced baby food is a great example. If you get bombarded with sugars at an early age, you can develop obesity and diabetes during early school years. Today it is quite possible to give children and teens adult-onset diabetes. In other words, it is possible to give them an illness that used to take fifty or more years to develop. Humans sure know how to conquer nature!

But this process can be reversed. If you have gotten sick by means of consuming way too much sugar than your body can handle, decrease your sugar intake and eat your way to health. I have received hundreds of reports of success stories. Soon, doctors will be the only people that are unaware of this health prescription . . .

Food for thought: Reflect upon why children today develop adult-onset diabetes, and why that was impossible 50–60 years ago.

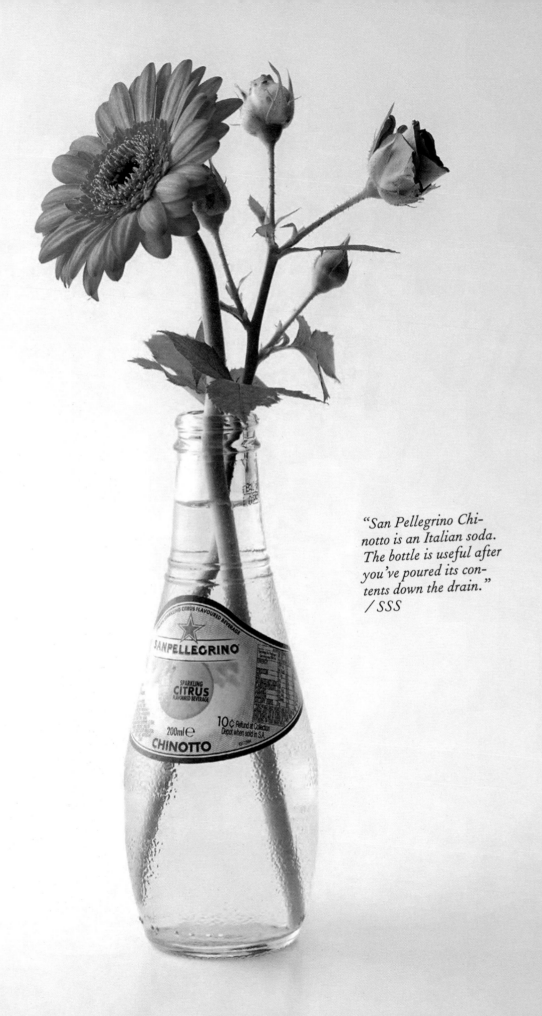

*"San Pellegrino Chi-
notto is an Italian soda.
The bottle is useful after
you've poured its con-
tents down the drain."
/ SSS*

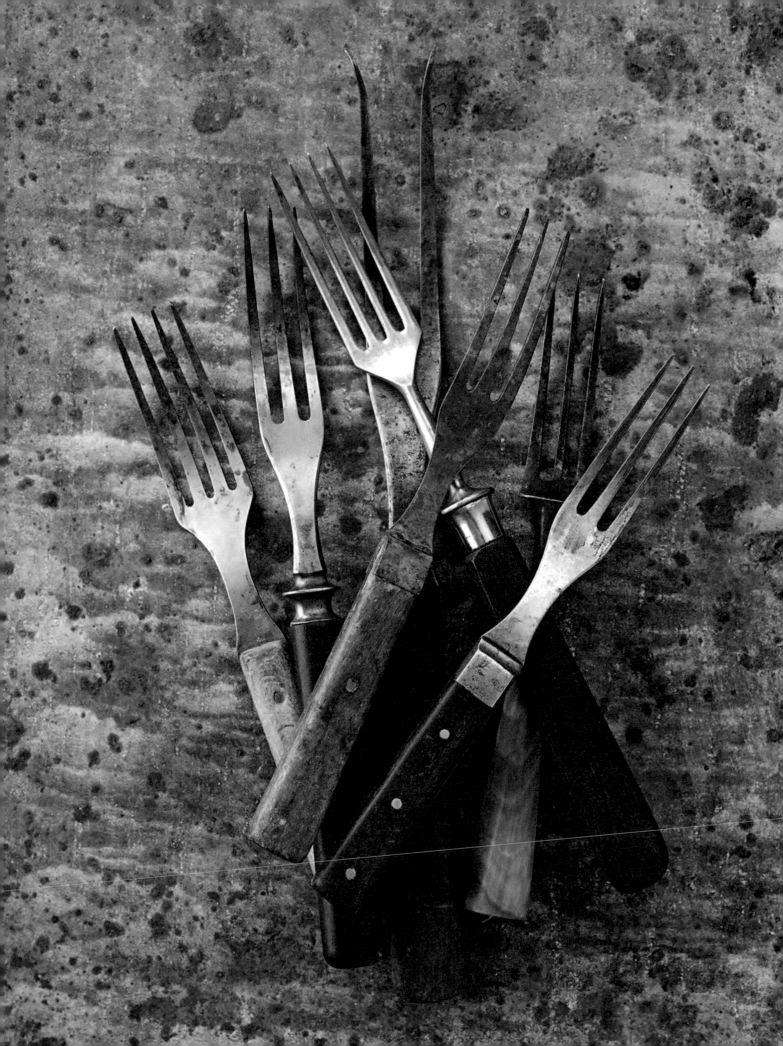

Eat your way to perfect health!

What happens to your health if you follow the new low-carbohydrate diet that I, and many others, have been developing since the year 2000? The diet is known for its natural produce, its large quantity of animal source fats, and few carbohydrates. Hundreds of thousands of Swedes and Norwegians have followed this diet (LCHF/GI-Zero!) for many years, and our experience with it has informed us of what is going on.

Diabetes (type 2/adult-onset diabetes) usually goes away in a few weeks. The blood sugar is stabilized and the insulin levels drop. You'll increase your healthy cholesterol levels, often to above two, and the triglycerides will decrease to below one. People feel healthier, they are able to decrease their medicine dose (no matter what type of medicine they are taking), and they lose weight. When we consume the foods that we were intended to eat, our body's natural ability to heal itself is triggered.

A lot of people that follow my diet are over sixty years old, and a lot of those people are severely overweight. They often suffer from metabolic syndrome, and according to my friends who are doctors, 2–4 percent of these high-risk patients suffer from a heart attack each year.

Can you guess how many thousands of heart attacks my readers and students have had out of the 100,000 followers in Scandinavia? The answer is zero! Not even those who have experienced heart attacks before starting the diet have had any new attacks. (It is common to die from a third heart attack.) With the LCHF/GI-Zero! diet, you don't get any heart attacks.

From this simple information, we can conclude that there is an easy cure for diabetes, heart attacks, infertility, intestinal problems, and obesity. Because it is impossible to patent this type of cure, no medicine manufacturers have any interest in spreading that knowledge, despite its potential to unlock the greatest medical revolution in our history.

Today, we know how to cure illnesses that kill millions of people in the West within a few weeks, using natural foods as medicine. Nothing more and nothing less. It was by chance that I rediscovered this method that people used to live by a hundred years ago. Today, there are several doctors in Sweden and Norway that have followed this diet for years and swear by it. Some of them even prescribe it to their patients as a way to regain their health. The most difficult challenge, though, is to stand up for your rights, since we are constantly met with resistance from people with higher titles who get paid huge sums to spread lies.

Simply put, you are responsible for your own health. This book is a good start to get you on the right track.

Index

10 9 8 7 6 5 4 3 2 1
Library of Congress Cataloging-in-Publication Data is available on file.

ISBN: 978-1-62087-783-8

Printed in the United States of America.